THE C LIST

Chemotherapy, Clinics, and Cupcakes:
How I Survived Colon Cancer

Rachel Bown

WATKINS PUBLISHING
LONDON

This edition first published in the UK and USA 2014 by
Watkins Publishing Limited
PO Box 883
Oxford, OX1 9PL
UK

A member of Osprey Group

For enquiries in the USA and Canada:
Osprey Publishing
PO Box 3985
New York, NY 10185-3985
Tel: (001) 212 753 4402
Email: info@ospreypublishing.com

1 3 5 7 9 10 8 6 4 2
Design and typesetting by Paul Saunders
Printed and bound in Great Britain by CPI Group (UK) Ltd, Croydon, CR0 4YY

A CIP record for this book is available from the British Library

ISBN: 978-1-78028-764-5

Watkins Publishing is supporting the Woodland Trust,
the UK's leading woodland conservation charity, by funding
tree-planting initiatives and woodland maintenance.

www.watkinspublishing.co.uk

To Lois and Joseph

In memory of Kate Needham
(1968–2013)

Contents

PART TWO

PART THREE

Foreword

Countless books have been written about the Big C – how to fight it, how to survive it, even how to accept it when the doctors say they can do no more, but *The C List* stands out from the crowd for it's originality and good humour.

Packed with sage advice, Rachel's lists, compiled during her cancer experiences, are funny, spot on and at times a little sad. After three major ops to remove the tumours from her bowel and liver, and eight months of chemo, Rachel has a lot to share.

The C List offers something for everyone affected by cancer, whether they are fighting the disease themselves or are caring for someone who is. The book's USP is that much of what Rachel wants you to know is presented in easy-to-follow lists, even if some of the lists themselves are plain bonkers!

Matthew Wright

2014

Prologue

What is a good list?

1. One that you nick and adapt as your own?

2. One that sticks in your mind long after you have read it?

3. One that you have scribbled on a beer mat or napkin?

4. One with some unusual *must-dos* and *must-nots*?

5. One that makes you laugh out loud?

6. One that gives you the sort of advice that saves your bacon?

Before you settle on your answer, let me give you a bit of background. You have picked up my book and might justifiably be thinking that you have stumbled across a list bore: someone who would leap into action and know just what to do when cancer was diagnosed, pushing organs and peace of mind aside.

In fact, you could not be further from the truth! I was neither organized nor prepared for this (is anyone when it comes to cancer?) and had to wise up pretty quickly. But thankfully, I had my A list of supporters and my endless lists for comfort.

If I am honest, I wrote those lists to help me create an illusion of control in what had become a chaotic, unpredictable life.

At the time, I feared that everything was going to slip through my fingers if I did not make lists. I also wrote them because I needed to quieten the deep-seated anxiety about not achieving or remembering what I set out to do: *like living long enough to teach my children resilience*, for example.

People asked me continually how I felt or dealt with what was thrown at me. So I thought it was about time I wrote it all down while it was still fresh in my mind and before it entered the realm of mythology.

And as I began this project of writing my story, I remember feeling the butterfly thrill of anticipation as I contemplated the silky sheet of paper in my new 'bought for cancer' moleskin book; the empty Microsoft Word page in front of me; even the back of my bank statement or any scrap of paper to hand.

I need to confess something at this stage: I do not limit myself to one list or form, as ideas tumble from my mind to my fingers while I type or scrawl across the page in unintelligible handwriting. No, I am certainly not that organized! (I once booked someone to organize me, and after a tour of my house and finding hair dryers in the same cupboard as saucepans, the person sent me a document on how she would declutter and organize me. Unfortunately, her number was on the document that I lost within days of its arrival, and so I was never able to book her to complete the job.) But I am energetic and full of hope, with a healthy love of anything or anyone hare-brained and absurd.

So bear with me as I take you through my story of being diagnosed with stage 4 bowel cancer at what I am now aware was the relatively young age of 45. I am a mother of two, with an interesting job, a lovely house in the country and more friends and family than I can fit standing side by side in said house. My life was as near perfect as I could wish for. I never wanted for anything, and my only worry was when my run of good luck was going to dry up.

But, and here's the important bit, despite the abrupt jolt to my peace of mind, don't be fooled into thinking that this is a misery memoir. Neither is it an 'I've got cancer, but let me tell you, it's the best thing that's ever happened to me' sort of book.

Instead, it is a wake-up call of what is important in life. It is about the daft and sometimes funny things that happen to people living with cancer, about the useful tips for making the best of it and about learning how to deal with your new menagerie of medics. Naturally, I found that most of the advice and insights fell rather neatly into lists that I could have really done with knowing before I started out on my ordeal.

I decided to call this book *The C List* as it occurred to me that apart from being a handy way to sum up any nuggets of wisdom I might have picked up from hundreds of sources along the way, I also wanted cancer to be demoted to the bit part it is, and for it not to loom so imposingly large in my life. It may have got hold of a sizeable chunk of my body, but I was damn sure it was not going to capture my mind. I was hell-bent on my A and B lists to continue and, come what may, to spend quality time with my dearest friends and family.

I was blindly oblivious and complacent about cancer. It could happen, or maybe it has happened, to you. I hope not, but if so, my wish is for this book to help you in some small way.

Here's my C list for starters! I had to shorten it as there really are a lot of things beginning with C …

C list for starters

1. Chaos
2. Comedy
3. Cuddles
4. Compassion
5. Cake
6. Chocolate
7. Champagne
8. Colonoscopy
9. Cancer
10. Colon
11. Catheter
12. Colostomy
13. Courage
14. Chemo
15. Crisis
16. Care
17. Clinic
18. Confidence
19. Carcinoma
20. Control

PART ONE

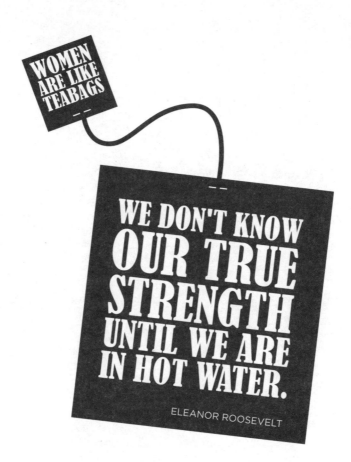

CHAPTER ONE

*

The Race for Life – or where it all began

> **To do**
>
> 1. Book doctor's appointment.
> 2. Remember to collect sponsorship this year.
> 3. Check if Cornish holiday apartment takes dogs.

I finished the 5k Race for Life on the Rye in High Wycombe in 32 minutes. Yes, I promised my mother and daughter that I would walk it as the doubling-up pain from somewhere unknown inside me was getting worse. But as I was dragging my body around the sea of pink again for the third year running in memory of my Auntie Naomi, who had died of bowel cancer at the age of 50 a few years previously, the emotion and adrenaline of the event overtook me, and I decided it would be gutless to walk (*just noticed how many synonyms for cowardice relate to the body: lily-livered, yellow-bellied, spineless, pigeon-hearted, cow-hearted, chicken-hearted, weak-kneed, having the willies*). It was also true that I would rather admit to a double homicide than concede to being outrun by my poor mother! So I ran sandwiched in between my 11-year-old daughter and my 65-year-old mother. I knew, as I finished, that something was wrong. You might sensibly wonder why it did not occur to me in a field hosed down with memories and experiences of cancer that I would also be carrying this disease. But all I can say is that humanity is divided by two great beliefs: it will never happen to me; and everything always happens to me.

I certainly belong to the 'it will never happen to me' camp. At the time of my diagnosis, I was a busy and working single mum with a son of 13 called Joseph and a daughter aged 11 called Lois. My daughter is uncannily like me, something which she welcomes on a pick-and-mix basis, but she is certainly more accepting of the chatty and blonde bit. My son, on the other hand, has more of his father in him and has suffered from anxiety all his life, resulting in many conversations held late into the night about the safety of me, the house, the dog, the car and just about anything that cannot be protected by a round-the-clock Special Forces squad posted outside our door. Lois doesn't see Stop or Caution signs and believes everything will get out of her way or will be less painful when she hits it, whereas Joseph would be far happier preparing for everything that can go wrong and alarming himself and me in the process.

I had never looked further ahead than the end of a sentence or felt I had a firm grip of anything in my life. My mind is just not wired like that. It works a bit like how I imagine flying a helicopter while mixing a cocktail would feel. Distracted, to say the least. But while I have never yet met or expected to meet anyone who felt in control and prepared for what was about to hit them – 'Cancer? Yep, I saw that one coming. Did not surprise me in the least' – I certainly could not have felt less ready or primed.

Keeping on the subject of minds for a moment, I had been drawn to a piece in the excellent book *Anticancer: A New Way of Life* by David Servan-Schreiber which puts forward a scientifically untested but nonetheless seductive theory. Schreiber's theory centres on whether it is possible for people to be psychologically predisposed to cancer. I have no idea if there is any merit in it, but there are psychotherapists who have worked with doctors in the field of cancer who have observed characteristics similar to my own personality traits. These are called Type C personality types and are about as far away from Type A or alpha females/males as you could get. So I took an inventory of my 'Top 5' personality rules and decided it was time for me to be a little more vocal about my fears and feelings and what I demanded from life.

List of my pre-cancer 'Top 5' personality rules

1. Don't do today what you can put off until tomorrow.

2. Confrontation must always be diffused with humour.

3. Making someone feel awkward is a capital punishment.

4. I obviously don't believe in capital punishment.

5. Don't grumble and carry on pretending everything is normal.

Before I turned up for my doctor's appointment a couple of days after the Race for Life, I allowed myself a spot of Googling and checked 'ulcerative colitis' which I thought explained my worsening symptoms. A friend of mine suffered badly with this condition and, from her descriptive updates, I thought this explained mine, too.

I still did not think for a minute I had cancer. If my auntie's death a few years earlier from bowel cancer had not alerted me to the possibility, what you might ask would? She had lost weight fast and continued the spiral downward. It was extremely painful to revisit or even talk about. In fact, I remember her illness being characterized by silence, only to be broken on occasions when we would see her at family gatherings looking vulnerable. Her husband and sons locked around her protectively.

We all cope differently in times of crisis, and Naomi chose to suffer quietly and with dignity. That is not to say she was not emotional, but she simply did not like talking openly about her feelings or symptoms. She certainly was not the blabbermouth I have always been (and continue to be!).

We were close, not just in age but in humour, too. She had a lively wit, and I have fond memories of driving in the car with her and her husband Guy, witnessing the sarcastic banter and good humour between them. They were my coolest relatives when I was growing up.

I had started a new job as Head of Marketing for a software company, and I remember talking a lot about her quick decline with a sense of disbelief. It was only my second experience of death. But it set off a domino effect, and our close-knit family was to suffer further deaths before I was finally diagnosed three years later. I was uncomfortable with the heat of a thousand light bulbs about any subject relating to death, so these years were one hell of a test.

My mother, however, was becoming more practised. She had lost her baby sister, Naomi, who was more of a daughter to her, followed quickly by her father, then her mother and, finally, her mother-in-law. She had nursed them all in their final years. No sooner had she buried them than my father was diagnosed with early-stage bladder cancer (which was luckily cured). Our family became accustomed to meeting up regularly at funerals.

Every year we would ask optimistically, 'Please let this year be gentler on us.' And we would pray that our most important decision in the coming year would be something like, 'Should we risk eating an apple without washing it first?'.

So I was not in denial or even living in wilful ignorance. No, it was the most common of reasons; while the flare-ups were irritating and, at times, painful, in no way did they equate in my mind to what it must feel like to have cancer.

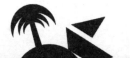

Smooth seas do not make skillful sailors.

African proverb

CHAPTER TWO

✳

At the doctor's

Three lesser-known facts

1. Cancer is not always painful and in any way obvious to the sufferer.

2. Bowel cancer is not just for the over-60s. I was not too young for bowel cancer: 2,000 of us under 50 will be diagnosed each year in the UK alone, and this category is growing fast.

3. Vegetarians can get bowel cancer, too.

I had visited my doctor twice before. The first time, I tentatively asked if bowel cancer could be a possibility and mentioned that my auntie had recently died of it and was 49 when diagnosed. My concerns were dismissed, and I was told that it was IBS (irritable bowel syndrome). When my symptoms showed no signs of going away and I was beginning to get worried about the number of times I was going to the loo, I went back again. This time, interestingly enough, I was told that it could be the early onset of the menopause. Apparently, the menopause can also play havoc with your bowels (filed away under 'Future evils').

When I turned up for the third time at my GP's, I did so without any hint of nervousness. But instead of seeing my regular doctor, there was a locum sitting in her chair. I remember being disappointed, thinking she did not know me, and this was going to be embarrassing discussing bowel movements with a complete stranger. How wrong I was – she was sharp, direct and asked me all the right questions. Questions I had avoided asking myself. And facts I would have shared less willingly than the pin number of my bank account.

She examined me, giving me a rectal examination and prodding along the length of my colon with her fingers, asking me what hurt and where. My stomach clenched and knotted, but I tried to focus on the absurdity of everything and moronically cracked jokes throughout the examination. Ms Locum did not join in. This was getting more uncomfortable by the minute.

She returned to her desk and began questioning me in depth while writing up a referral. I had answered yes to all what I now realize are the red-flag questions and was therefore an urgent case for hospital referral. Despite this, she was calm and composed.

'Right, I'm going to refer you for a colonoscopy which according to the government's targets needs to happen within 14 days.'

'But I'm going to Cornwall with my children in two days' time and will be away a week,' I complained.

Without looking up, she enquired, 'Do you need to go? Can you change your plans?'

'No, I really need to go. Can you just ask for my colonoscopy to be scheduled after I get back? Does it need to happen so quickly?'

I mean, I had already squandered a year since the first symptoms. Surely another week would not be a problem?

'Unfortunately, it doesn't work like that. The appointment has to happen within 14 days. If the appointment comes through for the week you are on holiday, I'll have to start the referral process again, and I wouldn't recommend delaying it any further.' She paused. 'Do you have any private healthcare? They may be able to be more flexible with dates. You could try and get an appointment as soon as you come back from holiday.'

I said a silent thank you, the first of many, to my company for including private healthcare in my benefits, and although I had regrettably turned down my one 'get rich quick but painfully' scheme, by adding critical illness cover to my company benefits, I was at this point deeply grateful that I had not also changed my mind on private healthcare cover. I did wrestle with my decision to choose private over the NHS, but the clincher was the speed and flexibility of my treatment options. The only downside I can now think of was the lack of a specialist nurse assigned to you to coordinate your care and spend time answering your questions – hence my obsessive need to research and write down everything!

Next followed a hectic few hours in which I told my mother, and we had the first of many conversations entitled 'What if ...' to prepare both of us, as I later realized, for the likely eventuality of cancer being discovered. Unlike me, my mother had obviously already considered this possibility and was calm despite what must have been her worst nightmare, with the recent loss of her baby sister from the same disease, still unbearably raw.

And then I hit the phones. What colorectal surgeons operate at the Chiltern Hospital? When are they available? I am ashamed to say that, at this stage, I did not think of checking their records or specialism, still not quite believing I would need them.

I found my surgeon, Mr H, more by luck than judgement as he was one of the few who was not on holiday in August and happened to be free the week after next. My father, however, not being one to trust luck, had read every paper tucked away down the back of the Internet referring to my surgeon and considered him an excellent choice. I booked the appointment and filed it under 'Unpleasant things to do when I come back from holiday'.

The important bit to remember is that your mother, father, siblings and children will go through worse fears than you and will feel helpless. It is your duty to put them at ease and raise a smile or two. This is not the time for wallowing in self-pity. As my friend Kate reminded me of some unsolicited advice she was offered when going through the same cancer treatment: 'Come on, love, wipe your tears dry and stop crying. We are mothers! So slap on your lipstick, pin a smile to your face and put on a killer pair of heels!' A good tip, although I quickly dropped the heels and lipstick bit.

List of questions every good doctor should ask

1. *Have your bowel habits changed in the last three months? For how long have you had these problems and have they lasted longer than three weeks?*

Yes, now that I come to think of it, there have been significant changes, and the problems have lasted for possibly a year or more.

2. *Have you fluctuated from diarrhoea to constipation?*

Yes, that's exactly what happened.

3. *Where is the pain?*

On the right-hand side. It actually has stopped me from sleeping on my side. The only comfortable place is on my back.

4. *Have you ever felt like you haven't quite emptied your bowels after each bowel movement?*

Yes, I have. I've never thought about it like that before, but definitely yes.

5. *How many bowel movements do you have? Especially at night? Do you often wake up needing to go?*

Yes, recently about five times a night on average. (Saying it out loud, I thought, you idiot, how could you have thought that this was normal?)

→

6. *Have you ever spotted blood?*

Yes, at least three times over the last year. But as it was not regular until recently, I did not think it was important.

(By now I was feeling very guilty and incredibly stupid for ignoring it. My poor children and family. IDIOT!)

7. *Have you unintentionally lost any weight?*

Yes, about half a stone while still loading enough carbs to sprint the length of Britain.

And now for the killer question:

8. *Is there a history of bowel cancer in your family?*

Oh hell, yes, my auntie died of it a few years ago. (I had mentioned this at least twice previously to my doctor.)

9. *How old was she when she was diagnosed?*

Forty-nine. Just four years older than I am now. (The sound of pennies dropping was deafening.)

Now, if any doctors are reading this, please underline this bit! Never rely on your patients to be open about what is going on in their bowels. It is like the adult equivalent of teenage boys attempting to buy their first condoms. If you cannot blurt it out in the first few minutes, you are likely to leave the surgery with a prescription for happy pills. Questioning us about symptoms in a matter-of-fact manner works much better, allowing us to answer yes or no without having to go through the utter embarrassment of discussing poo with your doctor! (If you are reading this in 2020, I sincerely hope this is no longer the case ...)

I had no idea that such a thing as the Bristol Stool Chart existed, but it would have been a useful aide-memoire. It certainly caused my dad to sweat and dab his brow at the shock of seeing so many 'jobbies' on a screen the first time he saw it.

Courage doesn't always roar.
Sometimes courage is the quiet voice
at the end of the day saying
"I will try again tomorrow".
Mary Anne Radmacher

CHAPTER THREE

*

Getting through the days before it all kicked off

I tried to pack my worries away underneath the holiday para-phernalia and busied the children ready for our week in the area we all pretend has more sun than the rest of England – beautiful Cornwall. I think at this stage my brain was running on parallel tracks: on one operating normally and practically and on the other making big decisions almost subconsciously. One of these was the realization that I did not want my partner of six years to come on holiday with us.

He had moved in with us about three years previously. At first, he appeared to be in his element, looking after a family with young children. However, cute little children turn into teenagers who have their own opinions and need space to grow and develop independence. And as time wore on, my partner's face often bore the expression of a man in a losing struggle with unknown demons, and this air of intensity hung over our house like a heavy cloud. There were to be constant rows between him and my son, and my personality type sucked this up and tried not to rock the boat or provoke any arguments; instead, I used what little energy I had to try and jolly everyone out of it.

My favourite coping mechanism has always been to descend into 'light-hearted nonsense', which, after the week glimpsing future hell, I needed more than ever. Call it escapism or denial if you will, but I knew I had a precious few days to get my head together before facing whatever lay ahead. The children were, and are, my number one priority, and I needed to spend all my waking and sleeping hours with them. It was also no secret that the relationship between Joseph, my eldest child, and my partner had now completely broken down.

This left me no choice but to find the strength to break it to him straight that things could not go on as they had.

It went something like this …

Ring, ring, answerphone: *Hello! I can't come to the phone right now. Please leave a message.* (I knew he was away for the night at a friend's house.)

Umm, bit of an awkward message … 'You're not going to like this, but let's be honest: things are not working out, are they? I really think we need some time apart to decide what to do, and I need to enjoy a week with the children on my own without rows or atmospheres. Sorry to break it to you like this, but that's how I feel.'

And then suddenly as it dawned on me that he would be back the day I was going away and my guts certainly could not cope with any more emotion, I added, 'Oh, and I'm going a day early so I can drop in on Liz on the way, which means I won't be here when you get back. It's probably easier for both of us this way.'

After I had plucked up the courage to talk to his answer-phone, I realized that like most things in life, thinking about doing something is often much worse than actually doing it. I wish I could remember this …

As we drove down the endless roads to Devon and Corn-wall, I found that conversation with the children flowed easily and freely, and we all felt like naughty schoolchildren escaping a headmaster as we sung along tunelessly to the radio. However, I recall the moment perfectly when we entered the moors and the songs faded into a Macmillan radio advertise-ment which I seem to remember was stating the fact that one in three people will get cancer. Cancer was now casting a net of fear over us all. I had to grab my chance. 'It's amazing what they can do for cancer nowadays,' I said, casually.

'If you got cancer, I would die,' Joseph shot back instantly.

'Of course you wouldn't. Cancer's not a death sentence anymore. Loads of people have it now and survive,' I lobbed back.

'Oh yeah? I bet. Don't believe you. Who do you know who has survived, then? Go on, give me names.'

'Errm, Mary from work, Phoebe's mum Kathy, my cousin Mindy …' Awkward pause. 'Loads, absolutely loads.'

'Are you going to get cancer?' Lois asked, tuning in to the conversation.

'Who knows? More and more people are getting it, but it's so much easier to treat and cure these days, so even if I did, I wouldn't be worried. Well, it would be a pain, of course, but we'd cope and I'm pretty fit.'

'Really?' said Joseph, less convincingly, and then: 'OH GOSH, MUM, DO YOU HAVE IT?'

'Who knows? I doubt it, I feel fine. Do I look ill? Stop worrying and look at that bloke over there going for a wee,'

I pointed, suddenly delighted to see the proud, wide-legged pose of the long-distance man traveller.

As I drove on, I tried to hide the cramping and stabbing pains in my abdomen. It felt a bit like contractions. When I was not being watched, I found that rocking naturally like I was in labour helped the pain.

Stopping over at Liz's was a good idea: sleeping in a big bed on my own, all cuddling up on the sofa watching *Whistle Down the Wind* and my car deciding to break down which meant I had to 'man' up and try and sort it out myself. When I say 'myself', I mean I had to find a garage and flirt my way into getting served and have the car repaired immediately. I am relieved to say this not only worked, but I drove away without even having to pay a penny! Needless to say, Joseph announced this was because 'the man fancied you, Mum!'. Anyone who so much as raises an eyebrow at me 'fancies' me according to Joseph.

The week away allowed me to have precious time with my children on my own. And looking back, I seemed to have rattled through the week as if attempting my own bucket list (not something that I normally subscribe to), doing every-thing from surfing and segwaying to coasteering and zorbing. The children seemed to grow during the week as if in prepara-tion, and their new maturity was gently reassuring. I almost expected to see them sitting there reading the *Daily Telegraph*, telling me to tuck in my shirt after ticking me off for running in the corridors or texting while I ate.

Things not recommended before embarking on a wrestle with the Sly Old Fox (aka cancer)

1. Trying to split up with your partner or having those 'difficult but overdue' conversations.

2. Zorbing down a hill in Cornwall letting go of your two children, causing you all to bounce at speed off the sides and concussing the lot of you.

3. Coasteering: squeezing into wet suits and tempting death by leaping off large cliffs into the sea.

4. Holidaying a long way away from any accessible hospitals or family in Cornwall.

Things recommended before embarking on a wrestle with the Sly Old Fox

1. Finding ways to drop cancer into conversations in an attempt to take out some of its future sting – courtesy of Macmillan radio ads which prompted a valuable chance for discussion and debunking the terrifying myths kids have in their heads.

2. Having lots of lazy nights and all sleeping in the same bed, with no schedule or rules.

3. Changing your 'Out of office' alert to 'Sorry, I am busy, please come back in a year or two or three'.

4. Doing all of the above on the 'Things not recommended' list if it makes your children happy.

I had avoided all contact with my partner while on holiday, so the return home was a nervous, 'tummy gone missing, presumed in Cornwall' sort of experience. I have always buckled at the first sight of tears and, after much begging, allowed him to stay and prove to me he could get on with Joseph. He had always wanted to look after me, but, at this stage, I just was not aware of the cost for the rest of the family.

* * *

Later that week I had my first meeting with my colorectal surgeon, Mr H. For future reference, we will call him the Siamese Cat owing to his inscrutability and calm and somewhat distant oriental mystique. Our first encounter was short, sharp and slightly uncomfortable. Still thinking I would be having a nice little chat about my medical history during which time I shall be reassured and leave feeling slightly embarrassed for wasting everyone's time, I was to come home disappointed.

After recounting the facts, the first warning that I was not about to be fobbed off again was when he asked me to lie on my side on the couch. With a nurse present, he began a procedure known as a flexible sigmoidoscopy. That's a camera up the bum for those not familiar with the term. It did not hurt much, despite the contents of a king-size airbed being pumped inside me to enable a better view, and it was over in minutes. He washed his hands and asked me to rejoin him at his desk. There was no eye contact.

'Well, I can feel a lump in your tummy. It could be poo,' he shrugged, 'but I can also see remnants of dried blood.'

I remember being struck that my surgeon was using the word 'poo'.

'Okay, could this be ulcerative colitis?' I asked tentatively. 'Or IBS perhaps?' I continued hopefully, not recognizing my own voice.

There was not even a moment's hesitation before he replied, 'No, definitely not. Nor any of the inflammatory bowel diseases, for that matter.'

Why was he so sure that it was not Crohn's disease, for example, I wondered?

'We will get you in as soon as possible and do a full colonoscopy to see what's going on.' He sounded impatient or maybe just somewhat frustrated that I had left it so long to seek medical advice. Who could blame him? I could have punched myself in the face at this point.

But this answer was not going to satisfy my sudden urgent curiosity, so I pushed him again for his suspicions and he clarified, 'I'm afraid we're looking at either a large polyp which can bleed or at bowel cancer. Polyps are early growths that often lead to bowel cancer. We will know more once I've examined you under sedation.'

Bummer. I felt like most of the remaining air was being knocked out of me.

'I need to organize a colonoscopy at another clinic.' He looked at his calendar and began explaining that it needed to be done as a matter of urgency.

'Right, I have another week off the week after next and was wondering …' I trailed off.

'No,' he stopped me dead. 'No holidays, no leaving the country and no future bookings of any kind, please. I will see you next Wednesday, and we will know more by then.'

* * *

Meanwhile, my doctor had called me back in for a blood test. I had no idea what for, but all of the sudden I was getting a lot of unwanted attention from the medics.

As it turned out, my surgeon totally dismissed the blood test my GP had ordered, for the following reasons.

List of things to be aware of when having a GP blood test

1. Liver and kidney function can appear normal despite having cancer.

2. CEA levels (these measure tumour levels in the blood) can also be unreliable in some people. For reference, anything above 5 *can* be suspicious, especially if it is on an upward trend over time. However, many things can affect CEA levels, and they range enormously from person to person. Mine were normal ...

3. CRP levels (inflammation levels) are also unreliable and can appear normal or give false positive readings.

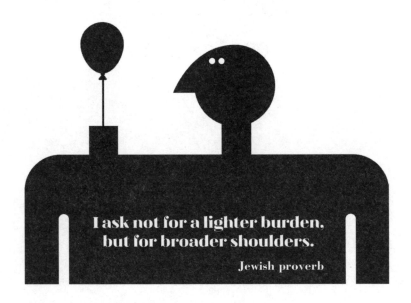

I ask not for a lighter burden,
but for broader shoulders.

Jewish proverb

*

CHAPTER FOUR

D-Day – or should I say C-Day?

Anyone facing a colonoscopy need not be afraid of the procedure. By far the most unpleasant part is the drinking of gallons of bowel preparation gunk to cleanse your colon. I am sure I do not need to explain the details of what happens next, but make sure you do not stray more than three paces from a loo! However, for me, unusually, nothing at all happened for the first half of the day. I phoned the Siamese Cat's secretary, a wonderful lady called Lesley, who was kind and professional. After talking through the lack of 'activity' with the consultant, she persuaded me to continue with the second dose. I spoke to my mother who sounded nervous. She feared my bowel was close to being totally obstructed and thought this 'inactivity' was further evidence of the seriousness of my situation. I had detected a note of concern in the secretary's voice as well which was a bit of a red flag.

However, on the morning of the colonoscopy I felt strangely calm and composed. I was given an enema, then sedated and taken into a room with a plasma screen. I prepared to go on a drunken simulated ride inside my large bowel.

Almost instantly the camera confronted a foreign object: I saw what appeared to be a butt-ugly tumour and heard the words, 'Take a biopsy and arrange an urgent CT scan'. I do not remember any pain or discomfort, which was odd as I was told this was likely if I had hairpin bends in my colon, so I enquired. 'That didn't hurt at all. I presume I must have gentle curves and not hairpins?' This was met with a gruff response from my surgeon who told me he would come and explain everything in a minute. He was not in the mood for chit-chat.

The next thing I remember was being back in my room, with the Siamese Cat showing me a picture of my tumour as if it were a scan of my unborn child. And with what felt like the brutality of a Canadian hunter killing a seal with a hakapik, he told me I had a 'nasty cancer' and that he was sending me down for a CT scan to see where else it might have spread. He added that he was not sure at this stage whether he would be able to operate.

I felt an instant wave of sickness hitting me. People describe severe shock as a physical sensation, and I now understand this. My chest began to constrict, and I struggled to breathe. The nurse raised my feet up above my head and stroked my hand to stop me fainting and parting company with the remaining contents of my stomach. My mum went white and was glued to the phone, calling relatives, starting with my brother. My dad and my partner were shell-shocked.

The nurse gently told me to drink a milk-like fluid over the next hour and explained that I would then be wheeled down to the CT department. When I'm in shock, I act even more daft. I was in utter shock and turned OTT silly. I sat by the door and let people in and out, joking about our fashionable attire. I joked with the operator as I passed through the doughnut-shaped scanner ...

I scanned the radiologists' faces for knowing signs; they were unbearably kind. Surely there was not any more bad news to come? I was told to return the next day to see my surgeon for my results.

We left and stopped at the pub on the way home, ordering a round of brandies. My father refused as he does not like brandy, but we all bullied him into downing one. Somehow my dad drove us back home. And with the hunger of condemned men we all ate Chinese takeaway and slept over at mine, courtesy of sleeping pills.

* * *

I am told there are four phases to dealing with cancer: diagnosis; waiting for the test results; treatment (operation and chemo); and the period following treatment or remission (in other words, the rest of your life).

It appeared that I was going to rattle through the first two phases in a matter of hours. While I am grateful I did not suffer the extreme anxiety of waiting for results, I think the speed in which my life changed caused such shock that it took me many months to process it.

Before I became personally acquainted with cancer, I always had had a ghoulish curiosity about how people felt when they were given a shocking or terminal cancer diagnosis. I read avidly on the subject, almost in an effort to cram in any information I could find should I ever be called upon to take a shot at the Sly Old Fox myself. Needless to say, at the moment when I was required to 'take an aim', my arm shook and I was unable to prepare myself for the kill. But this is how I remember feeling when instantly plunged into survival mode.

List of typical reactions to the shock of a cancer diagnosis

1. Your brain will attempt to protect you by shutting down very quickly. As you only have a small window initially to 'hear' information, consultants often may appear brutal or direct.

2. You may not want to know your prognosis immediately.
(I was terrified of accidently overhearing or reading something before I was ready to hear it.)

3. You might feel faint.
(I felt like a drunk who had stood up too quickly.)

4. Being indoors can feel repressive and claustrophobic.
(I needed to get outside and breathe deeply.)

5. You will struggle to make simple everyday decisions and probably need your family or friends around you to take over in the beginning.

6. You will not be able to deal with anyone else's pain *initially* and need to see people coping – or at least hiding their worst fears from you.

➔

7. Your mortality will hit you hard, and you will struggle to think about anything else.
   (I thought I was going to die quickly once I heard the word 'cancer'.)

8. You want people to stop loving or needing you, so it matters less to them when you are gone.

9. Death can become a preoccupation. (I was terrified that my parents would die before I was going to and there would be no one to look after the children.)

One piece of advice I wish I had followed was to avoid the Internet. But if you do want or need to find out more about your illness, trust the charity sites. They are accurate and helpful. I found three charities – Bowel Cancer UK, Beating Bowel Cancer and Macmillan – particularly invaluable and devoured all the information I could over the coming weeks and months.

* * *

The next day I returned with an even larger support team, this time including my younger brother, David. More chairs were called for. We were ushered in. My legs began to twitch as I tapped my feet constantly under the desk.

I will try to describe the Siamese Cat as the manner he broke the news to me caused me to want to leg it, for fear of hearing even worse news. The best way of painting a picture of him *at the time* was to visualize the sort of man who looked silently alarmed as if discovering his trousers were lined with the venom of a box jellyfish. The threat of sudden death meant he had to avoid any expansive gestures or expressions and so remained motionless and inscrutably still. I had not yet learnt that this disguised a deeply caring nature and an obsessively hard-working and talented surgeon. First impressions are not always right. I now trust this man with my life, and he has relaxed considerably with me as my treatment has progressed. I was so focused on my unravelling mind that I did not stop to think how difficult it must be to give life-altering news to your patients. Or how disappointing it must be to have to try and reverse damage that might have been avoided so easily in the first place.

However, I do think he had been absent on the week (presumably doing a double shift doubling as the Grim Reaper) when med school trained future doctors in the art of gradual disclosure.

He opened up my scans on his computer and angled the screen in my direction.

'You can see it's here in your bowel' – stop for dramatic effect – 'and we also think it's in your liver which, I am sorry to say, means it's secondary, or advanced.' He paused again, accompanied by the sucking-in of cheeks and the shaking of head.

'*And* it also looks like it's in your lymphatic system. As you can see from this scan, these lymph glands look enlarged, which means it could also be anywhere else in your body at this moment.' This was accompanied by more sighing and head shaking.

I could see bits of 'non-me' in my bowel and my liver. It did not seem conceivable that all this was going on inside me undetected for months, maybe years.

This news was brutal, and I was unprepared for the scale of my cancer as well as the speed of disclosure. Since then, the lack of trust in my body and any foresight I might have had about being ill has stayed with me. I am deeply mistrustful of my body now. I scarcely rely on it to go to the bathroom unaccompanied!

'I am sending you for an MRI scan now to get a detailed picture of what's going on in your liver,' he continued. Blast. The Siamese Cat had cut short my future. By how much I did not yet know, but from his demeanour and the information he gave me, I feared my 'Best before' date was fast approaching. There was nothing, no glimmer of hope, to counter these fears or to put anything in perspective. It left me 'hanging' and created the deepest fear imaginable. My father helped my mother out. I don't remember us speaking, but she told me that my face had turned to granite as I listened and watched with uncharacteristic concentration.

It seemed to me that my brain was appearing to slow down time, and I filed and remembered important facts, conversations and environments with clarity and colour, while jettisoning anything unnecessary.

I can remember the disappointing cold and greyness of the English summer as I waited alone for the MRI scan in a mobile unit in the car park outside the hospital. I fumbled with my Rescue Remedy and could not stop shivering. A nurse offered me a blanket, but it did not help. I was ordered to undress and to slip into a hospital gown. My fingers were incapable at that moment of undoing my clothes and bra, so the nurse helped me. Any last vestige of comfort was scattered on the floor as I climbed onto the scanner bed.

I asked for music, and after much searching for a CD, she put on Liszt. I still cannot listen to him to this day. Those 45 minutes were the loneliest I had ever encountered, and I had never felt so afraid.

I was injected with some substance into my arm. Headphones were put on, and music was piped into my ears, only interrupted with requests to hold my breath for 40 seconds at a time. I am relatively fit (yes, I realize the irony of saying this), but not having first trained as an oyster diver, I struggled and wondered how a smoker was able to hold his or her breath long enough to detect lung tumours. I prayed my liver was clear. I bargained. I pleaded with God, all to no avail.

* * *

The next day when I was out walking with my family, my surgeon called. I nearly dived into the bushes.

'I just wanted to let you know that your lungs are clear. And I am going to operate on you next Wednesday.'

What relief! Up until that point I was not at all sure they could do anything for me. To be honest, I was not even aware there was a threat to my lungs, but I now had the information I so needed. I was going to be treated! What my poor tired neurons made of this new piece of news was beyond me at that point.

The full MRI results were due back in a couple of days, and I was then going to hear whether I had stage 3 or stage 4 cancer and whether it had spread to a distant site and narrowed down my survival statistics further. I knew the significance of these results; however, I had come to the conclusion that I could not face going back to see the Siamese Cat to hear my prognosis.

Panic had set in, and so I phoned up my surgeon's lovely secretary to let her know that I could not face seeing him again. I would rather not know yet, especially if I was going to have a major operation the following week. So it surely was not necessary to see him? She was clearly a bit stumped to be talking on the phone to an ostrich! It did not help that the sand in my mouth was obscuring my speech.

'Well, I'm afraid it *is* necessary,' she pointed out. 'If you yourself don't feel up to it, then could you please send someone in your place to speak to Mr H?'

I was still convinced I needed complete radio silence so that I could focus on my immediate horizon: next week's op. I thought my fragile thread of hope would disappear if I received any further setbacks. So off went my brother to face my worst fears for me. I tried to keep myself busy. My cousin Sharon and Auntie Carol had come down to visit and took me for a walk in the woods to distract me. They were great company, and despite everything, we laughed. But I clearly had not thought things through. No news in this case was obviously going to be bad news! Would my brother have kept silent if he knew my liver was clear?

It took less than a nanosecond to get my answer when they returned. My brother's face said it all, but he still made an attempt at being positive. Bless him.

'Well, it's okay, just the same as we knew. No new "news".'

'So it's in my liver?'

'Yes, but only a little bit, and we knew that anyway, so it doesn't change anything.'

What really went on in that room, and how many times David practised the air of unaffected worry on the way home, I will never know.

Meanwhile, the Siamese Cat had phoned to reassure me, 'You are still young and you have young children, so we are going to be throwing everything at you!' This sounded more like a threat, but I smiled, said thank you and heard the sound of the klaxon. We are off!

I was too shocked at the time to face or question my surgeon too much, but I have since rerun the conversation in my head a number of times, and here are some of the questions I asked the Siamese Cat ...

List of questions to ask your surgeon

1. *What is the stage of my cancer, in TNM format?*

'T' stands for grade of tumour: 1–4 depending upon the size and reach of the tumour – for example, if the tumour has penetrated through the bowel wall. 'N' stands for lymph node invasion (0, 1 or 2 for severity).

'M' stands for number of metastases (spread to other distant organs).

(My cancer was T4N2M1. Which meant the tumour had broken through the bowel wall into numerous lymph nodes and had travelled to a distant organ, in my case the liver. I have no intention of bidding for this as a number plate just in case you were wondering ...)

2. *Can you tell if my cancer is fast or slow growing?*

Bowel cancer is usually one of the slower-growing cancers. Your surgeon will be able to tell you if you will have a series of scans weeks or months apart; otherwise, it may be tricky to be certain.

➡

---

3. *Do you have a surgical speciality for my cancer type?*

Ideally, you want surgeons with specialist knowledge of your cancer. (This is not always possible if you are admitted as an emergency.)

4. *Can you do the surgery laparoscopically (by keyhole)? And if so, is this the safest for getting a good look around?*

With a laparoscopy, recovery time will be much quicker.

5. *Will you perform a pelvic lymph node dissection?*

(I have read that at least 12 lymph nodes need to be examined to accurately stage colon and rectal cancers. I had 19 lymph nodes taken out, and 7 were found to be cancerous.)

6. *What are the chances that I will have a temporary or permanent colostomy? And if so, what type of colostomy will I have?*

Check with your surgeon if it will be a loop or end colostomy. This will depend on the position of your tumour. (Mine was an end colostomy.)

7. *How many of these operations do you do a year?*

8. *Can you do the operation first thing in the morning?*

As per my own online research, I have read about

➡

studies showing that morning surgery is less likely to go wrong.

9. *Statistically, what is the success rate for the operation and how does this compare with your op rates?*

10. *How long is the operation, including the period for the anaesthetic and the recovery room?*

    Your family will be counting every one of those minutes. Make it easier on them.

11. *Do you need to do this procedure immediately? What are the consequences of delay?*

    You may want an extra few days to do some research or even get a second opinion if you are unhappy with any of the answers.

In case you also have a liver tumour:

12. *Do you need to remove the liver tumour before you remove the bowel tumour?*

    There are different schools of thoughts here and many factors to understand: number of tumours, size, position and speed of growth.

13. *What level of pain can I expect after the operation?*

14. *Do you recommend an epidural or a morphine pump?*

➡

15. *Who can I call if I have any questions or concerns during my recovery?*

16. *Who will be coordinating my overall and follow-up care?*

17. *Who will explain my pathology (lab test results) to me?*

18. *What is my prognosis based on your current statistics?*

   You may not want to ask this question and prefer to be left in the dark. Also, statistics do not give you the real picture. You will be quoted the median. I took this to mean there will be people at either end of that curve that buck all trends and I was fully intending on being on the end of that tail.

19. *Are there any clinical trials for my type of cancer? Do you recommend I get on one?*

20. *Are there any specialist hospitals for my type of cancer?*

It always seems
impossible,
until it is done.

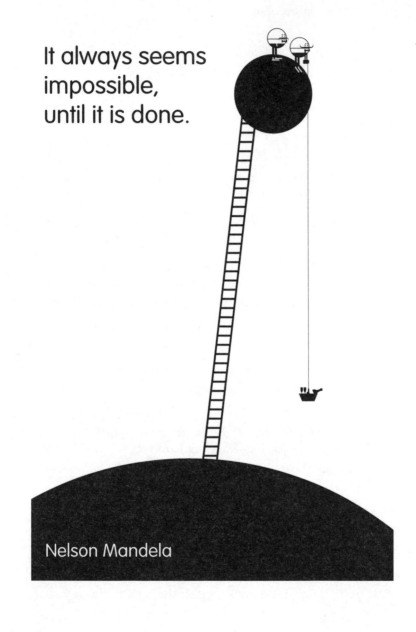

Nelson Mandela

CHAPTER FIVE

✳

Telling the children

I could not delay the arrival back home of my children any further. I had sent them away on the day of the colonoscopy in case I needed to get my head around any facts first. I did not want them to be a witness to the shock and the initial lack of facts, aware that fears grow to fill those gaps of knowledge.

But the children were now asking to come back home. Joseph was staying with Jenny, my best friend, and her son, Matthew, who was also, rather neatly, Joseph's best friend; Lois was staying with her best friend Livvy.

I knew this was the hardest thing I would ever have to do in my life, and I wasted no time making small talk. Your foremost instinct is to protect your children, but I also knew they would cope better if I was honest from the outset and kept them informed every step of the way. I knew my son would be suspicious that I was keeping something from him. However, I was also aware how much he and my daughter could take on board initially, so I tried to protect them with the gradual disclosure method.

Joseph and Lois arrived home in a jumble of noise and bags, immediately hugged me and said how much they had missed me. They began showing me things they had bought. I cut them short. I had to. I kissed them both, said I had something to tell them and asked them to come upstairs into my bedroom. The rest of the family stayed downstairs.

They both froze and cried out, intuitively aware that their lives were about to change, forever. Why were they being taken upstairs? What were they about to hear? I was not behaving like their mum.

There are no words to describe the next hour all three of us went through as I tried to break the news to them as carefully as I could. Joseph sobbed and held on to me as if his strength alone could save me. Lois went mute and moved away from me to the bottom of the bed, distancing herself from the horror that she must have felt. She picked at the quilt with her fingers and avoided my eyes or arms. After an age, she asked to go downstairs.

On a few occasions over those first few weeks, Lois asked, 'Can we please not talk about it?' as she obviously tried hard to shut it out. I was guided by her and Joseph's reactions and reacted instinctively. You can look at the following list and try and follow as much advice as possible, but, ultimately, you will know your own children best, and know how and what to say. Of course, the amount of information and the way you break it will differ enormously depending upon their age. Try not to over-rehearse what you will say to your children: natural and honest is best. You will have plenty of time to repeat again and again the information over the weeks and months ahead.

Macmilllan, Cancer Research UK and BUPA all have excellent advice on their websites on how to talk to children about cancer.

Tips on how to tell your children that you have cancer

1. Explain clearly, calmly and be as specific as you can. (I drew a picture to help them visualize where my cancer was. It will replace pictures they may inaccurately have in their head.)

2. Tell your children what the plan is to remove or treat the tumour and when this will begin. (I told mine, 'It's a little ball of cancer, and it's here in my bowel. Luckily, I can have an operation, and they can cut it out and join the bits of my bowel back together again.' They still remember those words and the picture I drew to this day.)

3. Explain to them what cancer is if they are able to take this in. Also explain what chemo or radiotherapy is if you are going to have it.

4. Tell them it is not contagious. They cannot catch it. (I was reading about the shocking number of children who believe you can catch cancer only recently.)

5. If you are having an operation, tell your children how you will feel and the likely recovery time so that they are not shocked when the time comes. (I told mine it might be better not to come and see me for the first day or two as I did not want them to see me surrounded by all the scary medical tubes.)

→

6. Tell them that the treatment will make you ill, but it is the treatment, not the cancer, that is having this effect. Explain that the treatment is necessary to make you better.

7. Tell them about people you know who have survived this and are doing well. Give them names and stories to make it more real.

8. Be as honest as you can. Don't lie or make promises, but also don't burden them with everything immediately. Gradual disclosure works for children, too.
(I chose not to tell mine about my liver immediately as I did not have a plan yet for removing it, and I felt at the time it was better to introduce this later once they had seen that I had survived one operation.)

9. Tell your children there was nothing anyone did to cause the cancer.

10. Let them know that their schools will be told immediately so that they can leave a lesson at any time if they feel they need space or comfort.

11. Let them tell their best friends when they are ready so that they can talk to them in their own time and way.
(My children were so lucky with their friends, Lauren, Livvy and Matthew, and have built even closer bonds this year.)

➡

12. Let your children know that you will answer any questions they have, especially the tough ones like 'Are you going to die?'

13. Give them suggestions on things they can do to help and support you so that they feel involved and actively can take part in your recovery.

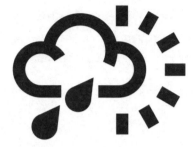

Weather: Whatever

Life is not about waiting for the storms to pass. It's about learning how to dance in the rain.

Vivian Greene

CHAPTER SIX

✳

The op

'I'm expected to make a decision on rerouting my gastrointestinal system and having it poke through my stomach in how many hours exactly?' I was looking at the Siamese Cat in disbelief.

Let me get this straight. Before my big day, I had just enough time to squeeze in one more big decision. Option one: when my tumour, which is low down in my bowel near my rectum, has been cut out, there is an option to join the two sections of my bowel back together again. Option two: I could choose to opt for a stoma and for the surgeon to reroute my large bowel, stitch it to a small opening on the left-hand surface of my stomach and seal up the other end to my rectum. This will mean that I will have a colostomy bag to attach to the stoma. Tell me again: why would I choose option two?

Why indeed? Well, according to the Siamese Cat there is a small risk that, when rejoining the bowel after the cancer has been removed, the join will leak. If this happens, it is serious and septicaemia will probably set in. This is life threatening, and you will have to undergo an emergency operation. But here is the shocker: if this happens, chemo or any further operations will be delayed for up to six months, while your body recovers. In my case, with two operations and chemo scheduled ahead of me, my surgeon did not want to delay treatment as it could skew my chances between survival and death.

I paced around the garden and concluded that while the risk was small, if I was unlucky enough to be in the option one category, it could be game over for me. Whereas in the other camp, the only risk was to my vanity, body image and, *possibly*, relationships. Put like that there really was no option. If having a bag could reduce the risks of me dying, then I just had to get on with it and accept it. I stress that this was two days after I had been given the diagnosis of advanced bowel cancer, and I now had just 48 hours to make my decision.

I told the Siamese Cat that I was opting for a colostomy bag. But I could have thumped him when he seemed shocked at my decision and wondered how I had arrived at this choice! In hindsight, I now realize that he may have overplayed the risks. Still, the decision was out of the way, and all I had to do now was to prepare myself and my children for what it would feel like to be the proud owner of a new bag. Mama's got a brand new bag! Funky. Take that, James Brown!

Thankfully, there were two people who helped me accept this decision, and I owe them a big debt. One of them was Ruth, a dear new friend who was campaigning big time in the media at that time to find a surgeon to operate on her. Despite this and her, at the time, very poor prognosis, she was massively encouraging about the stoma and told me it would be fine. I would adjust quickly and easily. It was not important and would not bother me at all once I had got used to it. And as far as anyone else was concerned, I should just tell him or her to think of it like a big plaster. She had modelled for Ostomy Lifestyle (a specialist help and support charity for stomas) to help break the taboo of having a stoma and looked absolutely beautiful. The decision was made. Goodbye, flat tummy. Hello, accessories under my clothing.

Unfortunately, there is still much secrecy around as to who has a colostomy bag, which you can get for Crohn's disease or ulcerative colitis as well as for bowel cancer. It would be wonderful if we could break this last taboo, but for the moment I was comforted by some famous names who had shared my new plumbing design – Napoleon Bonaparte, the Queen Mum, Fred Astaire, Bob Hope, Virginia Ironside …

* * *

7.30am. I arrived at the hospital and buzzed the barrier to be let in. 'Hello, can we help you?' the receptionist asked. 'Yes, Big Mac and chips please,' I nervously called out. The barrier went up and we were in.

I was shown to my room, began unpacking what little bits and bobs I had hurriedly put into my bag and stared ominously at the paper knickers, support stockings and obligatory backless gown laid out on my bed. This was no honeymoon, for sure.

The Siamese Cat arrived to get me to sign the consent forms and started to mark me up for the position of the stoma with a magic marker. 'Where do you wear your trousers? On the waist or below?' he asked, poised with the pen in hand. 'Eek, I have no idea,' I gushed. I had not expected this question! About here, I motioned, and a big old black dot was drawn on my stomach on the left-hand side about half way down. I immediately doubted my decision, but as the Siamese Cat did not look like he had brought some erasing liquid, I decided I had better live with it.

Not easing the pace of disclosure for a moment, he wasted no time in alarming me that it was 'possible, just possible', pinching his thumb and index finger together and creasing his face into a grimace, 'that we can reverse the colostomy bag one day'. 'Possible?' I gasped. 'I'm working on definite,' he shrugged. 'I'll attempt to do your operation by keyhole, but you do realize that if we find any obstructions, we will have to do open surgery.' 'Yes, I understand,' I said, getting the gist of this game of last-minute nerves. No, I won't sue or shout at you if I wake up looking like an extra on *Holby City*.

I was on my way now, no turning back. In a way, the speed from diagnosis to surgery was a huge benefit; by far the worst times are the days or weeks before you are on the treatment pathway. Once you begin, you can put all your energies into fighting back at this disease. But the downside is that it gives you far less time to deal with and process the shock. I know from my own and from friends' experiences that the shock lasts at least three months, so take it easy on yourself and slowly adjust during this period.

So, now fresh from my morning enema and with clammy hands, I was wheeled down to the operating theatre. I met my anaesthetist again and felt even less reassured than the first time. I was fortunate enough to have had my op and treatment done privately, but have come to the conclusion that private healthcare is charged out by the word: I can honestly say that the person responsible for keeping me alive during the operation did not waste a penny!

He asked the mental health-check question, 'You do realize

what you are here for?' I wished I had been as quick-witted as my friend Liz, who had said, 'Yes, of course, I'm having a baby.' (I am sure Liz won't mind me telling you that she was deep into her 40s by then.)

He gesticulated to me that I would be having an epidural block and motioned for me to sit up, lean forward and not move a muscle. By this time, adrenaline was pumping through my veins like the fuel injection in a McLaren, and I talked in rapid, nervous sentences. Needless to say, I was the only one. The needle going into my spinal column and the pushing sensation were painful, and I pleaded for more pain relief. Eventually I was stable enough to lie back down on the trolley.

At no point did I decide to fall in love with my anaesthetist – a common occurrence, I am told – as it was clear there would be no bedtime soothing words or gentle stroking of my hand. The door opened, and the God-like presence of the Siamese Cat suddenly appeared, with the theatre lights shining behind him and only his outline visible. Clearly, my anaesthetist suffered from the same sense of shock at the surgeon's unexpected appearance as I did and uttered 'Mr H!' as if caught having a sneaky nap with his patient before speedily pumping the anaesthetic into my canula without even counting down from ten. I stuttered 'Oh' and fell deeply asleep.

* * *

Some hours later I awoke coughing and a nurse appeared, saying, 'Well done, Rachel, you are in recovery.' Instantly, a wave of euphoria followed by sickness washed over me. I wanted to kiss her. 'Sick,' I muttered (not in the teenage sense, that would have been disrespectful). 'Okay,' she said and injected me with a strong anti-sickness drug. 'Did I get away with keyhole?' 'Yes.' More blissful relief. I lay for some time in a morphine cloud but with certain senses heightened. Hearing is one of them, and I listened to the conversations between the recovery staff and the ward nurses to bring me back into focus. The clock said 2pm. 'Listen, I know you haven't had lunch, but neither have we. No, I can't wait another half an hour.' This was repeated at least three times over the hour.

Bossy ward nurse must have won as the clock indicated 3pm when I arrived back in my room. I was allowed to sip a little water and my voice started to loosen up. I still had words to say, cut short by my anaesthetist, and boy, did I want to talk, awkward though it was with all the tubes and oxygen masks. But I was alive and drugged to the eyeballs! What utter bliss!

Sometime later the Siamese Cat arrived to talk to me. 'The operation went as expected. No more, no less. I have removed the tumour and also 19 lymph nodes,' he said. Is this good, I wondered? But I knew better than to fish for any positive news. So I nodded and said thanks. What else do you say to a man who has spent the last few hours inside your body?

I held off my children visiting until Day 2 when I hoped I would lose one or two of my tubes and look more mum like. Expect to be hooked up to drips, epidural (or morphine pumps), oxygen, a catheter, a colostomy bag, automatic blood pressure machines and machines attached to your legs, squeezing and releasing every few minutes. You certainly are not going to look your best, and you will not be able to give anyone a big cuddle without dislodging some tubes. But for some reason I thought it would be a capital idea (that was the morphine talking) for my mum to take a picture of me as proof I was alive and feeling good. I had no idea what I looked like, but suffice it to say, it did not reassure anyone! Still, I was amazed at how quickly this whole apparatus came down.

I have come to realize that a 'visit' to a hospital is prized above all things, and so armed guards were necessary to hold back the crowds wanting to peek at the patient.

After five nights in hospital, during which my room resembled the conservatory at Kew Gardens, I was sent home with bags of medicine to continue my recovery in familiar surroundings. My family were, and have been, my carers for this last year, and I have never heard them complain once.

I know it is often difficult to prepare for an operation, especially if it is an emergency admission, but I wish I had known a bit more, hence this next list.

List of things to be aware of after a major operation

1. You will be high on morphine or equivalent for Day 1 and 2 and probably be exhilarated to be alive.

2. You will crash on Day 3 or 4 (this is normal).

3. Your bowel does not like being touched and will sulk for days afterwards. This can be quite painful and you will experience feeling bloated. You will feel more comfortable after any wind has passed through.

4. You may feel pains in your shoulder afterwards caused by the air having been pumped into your abdomen.

➡

---

5. You will get little sleep with the noises from the machinery as well as nurses waking you every few hours for observations – take ear plugs!

6. Your surgeon will bully you into getting better by suggesting you should be leaving to go home far earlier than told/expected. This is normal behaviour. Anger will galvanize you into getting better more quickly.

7. You will receive a visit from a physiotherapist who will bully you into moving. This will seem impossible on the first day, but you will be surprised how quickly you improve.

A HERO

IS AN ORDINARY INDIVIDUAL WHO FINDS THE STRENGTH TO PERSEVERE AND ENDURE IN SPITE OF OVERWHELMING OBSTACLES

CHRISTOPHER REEVE

⁂

CHAPTER SEVEN

My treatment plan

There is the hard way to cope with a cancer diagnosis or the slightly less hard way …

Having tried to do this the hard way, I would be negligent if I did not offer you some insight into trying to avoid this and give you my tips on how to cope with a cancer diagnosis.

1. Forget certainty
There is no such thing as black or white with cancer. So knock that notion on the head. Embrace grey. And avoid anyone who swears by predictions: anything can happen, and things often change, sometimes for the better.

2. Get as many facts as you can
See List of questions to ask your surgeon, page 36.

3. Be prepared
Prepare yourself for changes to your physical appearance.

The more you anticipate this in advance, the less of a shock it will be when you have to confront these changes.

4. Get used to paranoia

Every ache will herald a fear of spread, progression or re-occurrence. This is as normal as the sun rising in the morning. Don't beat yourself up about it!

5. Get used to hospital visits

You will be popping into hospital as regularly as you are used to popping into the supermarket. Your weekly schedule will revolve around it.

6. Keep it simple

Try and live as simply as you can. Get off the treadmill. Think of the saying by the economist Tim Jackson: 'We spend money we don't have on things we don't need, to make impressions that don't last on people we don't care about.' Cancer is the best excuse you will ever have of getting rid of things you don't need and embracing the simplicity of living in the present. Taking one day at a time is all you can cope with when your future is uncertain.

7. Connect

This may not be for everyone, but it helped me. I connected with people who were going through the same as I was go-ing through. Join Twitter and Facebook groups or forums if you are into social media. There is a lot of support and information out there from like-minded individuals. You will not need to explain things, those in the same boat as you will just get it. However, there is a dark side, and you may not be ready to hear the sad stories yet. So protect yourself if it all gets a bit heavy. And take regular 'SM/social media' breaks!

8. Live healthily

For any cancer, it is important to eat as healthily as you can and to find ways to reduce stress. Dog walking, acupuncture and meditation helped me get through.

9. Love and be loved

There is nothing more soothing. Never underestimate the power of compassion. Research shows that you can train yourself in cultivating self-compassion that can give you the courage to overcome your own fears. Be kind to yourself and others. Take good care of yourself with plenty of rest and exercise if you can bear it. Surround yourself with people you love and try to find some balance in your life, however difficult.

10. Find your coping mechanism

Mine was humour and blogging. It kept me focused on finding amusement even in the most hidden of corners.

11. Have fun

Remember how to have fun! Dust off your imagination and think of things you would love to do. Choose easy things to do that are not dependent on time.

And most importantly:

12. Take one step at a time

I knew I had to face two major operations, one minor op, learning all about living with a stoma, at least six months of chemo, two clear CT scans and one clear colonoscopy before I could even think about a reversal operation and getting back to normal. Don't let your head rush ahead with you! Tick off each big step and celebrate it. My family brought me a charm bracelet, and after every operation, scan and chemotherapy session they gave me a charm to celebrate getting through it.

* * *

Here I was now, about to add a laid-back oncologist to my list. The next big thing to tick off in my treatment plan!

About a week after being sent home from hospital, my surgeon arranged an appointment with my oncologist who was now taking over my care. Dr W – or the Cheshire Cat, as we will call him – had an altogether different bedside manner than his colleague, the Siamese Cat.

He looked like the sort of man who was fighting a losing battle with narcolepsy, but to avoid detection, he stretched his mouth into a wide smile and tilted his head slightly to one side. All the same, he exuded an air of calmness and absence of panic, and I felt gratefully soothed by this.

We went in mob-handed with tape recorders, with my father speedily recounting to me some positive survival stories for reassurance. As we were unsure of what we were going to hear, we wanted to keep up our spirits. To be honest, I was relieved to finally get into the Cheshire Cat's office as my father's growing anxiety had seen him picking off patients in the waiting room in search of light conversation. One man could not have buried his head any further into his news-paper, but my dad was not to be deterred and launched in with 'Capello?', presumably because the man bore a minute passing resemblance to Fabio. That is if you were driving at 90 miles an hour and happened to glance over at him driving at a similar speed in the opposite direction.

The Cheshire Cat took us all in his stride and gave me a warm welcome before asking, 'So, tell me what you have been told so far.' I recognized this instantly as the idiot's bravado test. Are we dealing with someone who thinks they will be back at work by the end of this consultation and can cure it with a bit of something they read about in the *Daily Mail* this morning, or have they done their homework and are likely to take longer than their allotted time asking heaps of questions? I hope I inched towards the latter.

Obediently and nervously I rolled off, 'I have just had an operation to remove the tumour in my large bowel. It also looks like the cancer's in my lymph, and I have mets in my liver which I hope will be removed.'

'Yes, well done! That's about it. You have a tumour in your liver, but we have removed the bowel tumour and also 19 lymph nodes, and have found cancer in seven. We will need to start chemotherapy in a couple of weeks as soon as you are strong enough after your bowel operation. You will be on Oxaliplatin as an infusion every three weeks, together with two weeks of chemo tablets called Capecitabine – two weeks on and one week off. We will run this for three months, then scan you again and, hopefully, operate on your liver and mop up afterwards with another three months' chemotherapy.' And breathe.

'Am I likely to suffer side effects from the chemotherapy?'

'Maybe, it's possible, but maybe you won't. Everyone is different.' Huh?

Well, this was going to be one hell of a party and I would be a fool to turn down an invitation like that!

So off we went, me with my nice new brochure of side effects to study and a feeling of hope. And the Cheshire Cat could not have been any nicer if he were carved out of Swiss chocolate!

List of questions to ask your oncologist

1. *Why did you choose this particular chemo regime for me? Are they the latest and most successful drugs? Do you have any studies to back this up?*

2. *Can I have a list of the side effects and possible reactions to this chemo regime?*

3. *How many antiemetic drugs are there available to me?*

   (Antiemetic drugs are effective against nausea and vomiting.)

4. *Are there any clinical trials I could benefit from?*

5. *Can I be KRAS-tested to see if I will respond to this particular regime?*

   (You might want to ask this question if your cancer has metastasized. The test shows whether the KRAS gene in your cancer is mutated (changed) or non-mutated (wild type). It is a gene that contains the code for developing a KRAS protein involved in cell growth and cell division. Apparently, about 40 per cent of people with colorectal cancer have a mutated gene. It is worth finding out if you can as it can affect the type of drug options open to you.)

6. *Do you practise integrated medicine? If not, do you have any objections if I follow a nutrition-based programme alongside my treatment?*

7. *How often will I see you?*

➜

In addition to these questions, I also asked my oncologist to recite the names of anyone he knew who had my type of cancer and treatment and was still alive after five years.

* * *

One of the toughest things is telling someone you love that you have cancer. And I had to do quite a bit of this in the first couple of weeks. Everything had happened so fast: a week from diagnosis to first major surgery. Despite this, it was amazing how many people wanted to come and see me immediately. I could have sold out the O2 Arena! At least I had some time to get my head around it, but my friends were hearing it for the first time and suffered from enormous shock and grief. This can do funny things to even the most erudite of people.

Sadly, most of us will have to face listening to someone telling us they have cancer at some stage in our lives, and it got me thinking how I have reacted in the past when people have told me they had cancer. Not well, I am ashamed to say. So, being on the other end of the conversation, I can now give you some help on how to react when someone tells you they have the big C.

1. *Listen*
Hold the person's hand, hug them and let them talk, talk, talk. I yacked on forever. Repeating information makes it easier to come to terms with what is happening. Be a good listener.

2. Be patient and wait your time

This is a really personal thing and you need to be prepared to watch and wait a bit – during the first few weeks after someone is diagnosed, there is a huge deluge of terrifying information for them to deal with. Cancer is a long journey, there will be plenty of time later to call or visit. Texting is better as the phone never stops ringing in those early days. Make sure you are clear that you don't expect a reply. This will take the pressure off.

3. Sort out your role in all this

You could offer to research information, such as positive case studies, chemo regimes, and so on. (Don't let your recently diagnosed friend trawl the Internet unsupervised – the things they read in those first dark weeks will worm their way into their brain at night!) You would save them time and energy by sharing useful information with their friends and family. Offer to shop and cook for them; take them out for coffees; keep them healthy: find out the best food to eat, the best supplements, any complimentary treatment, and so on. I have been incredibly lucky as my family took on all these tasks for me.

4. Hide your fear

Whatever you feel, try and hide it. That is easier said than done, I know, but you want to avoid letting your fear bounce back on the person who is ill.

* * *

As I walked into the bright and airy reception of the Churchill, a specialist cancer hospital in Oxford, the sight of cancer patients *en masse* hit me hard. It was as if I was witnessing my future stumbling groggily towards me. I wanted to run away. I felt that I did not belong there. I had a full set of hair, and my body did not betray any of what was going on inside it.

Despite the shock of facing up to what was about to happen to me, I liked the hospital. It had a nice feel about it. I was miles away from recommending it on TripAdvisor, but all was not lost.

My oncologist, the Cheshire Cat, had arranged for me to go there to have a PET scan which involved me being injected with a radioactive substance called fludeoxyglucose. It is a bit like receiving an injection of a liquefied chocolate bar left behind at the Fukushima plant! Apparently, this is the equivalent to the recommended limit of radiation that anyone working in a nuclear power station should be exposed to in one year.

The injection came in a plutonium casing, and it was injected slowly into my body over an hour. After that, I was told to visit the special loo as I would be radioactive and therefore could not use the main patient toilet. Very alarming!

Cancers are hungry for glucose, and so the PET scan picks up 'hot spots' that are most likely cancer; these scans also are used to check how much a cancer has already spread, and they are usually done after the initial diagnosis has been made by an MRI or CT scanner or, in my case, both.

Not the most relaxing way to spend an hour. I was cold and uncomfortable, but as a professional scan junkie by now, I took this one in my stride, too, despite worrying whether the cervical scare I had a few years earlier resulting in two cone biopsies had progressed (I was overdue for a check) or whether my 25 years of near constant mobile phone usage had caused any brain tumours. How would the medical profession deal with two primary cancers at the same time, I wondered?

A couple of days later a surprise call from the Cheshire Cat on the way back from a school meeting revealed the news I had not quite dared to hope for: the cancer had not progressed any further from the one tumour in the liver and lymph glands. I cried tears of joy and hugged my friend Jane, who had given me a lift to school and who cried along with me. A moment of real happiness and the exact moment I felt I could win this dust-up with cancer.

My surgeon decided to operate on my liver as soon as possible. The multidisciplinary meeting (MDT) had weighed up the odds and decided that chemo to stop further spread, followed by a liver operation, followed by further chemo to mop up, was riskier than delaying chemo for another six weeks or so while we got the little bugger out my liver first. So it was now all systems go for my liver resection. I did warn you that, with cancer, things can change dramatically from one moment to the next.

When I met my liver surgeon, Mr S (we shall call him Felix the Cat on account of him having a magic bag of tricks), to go through the pre-op checks and to question him on what it all meant, he casually dropped in that he would also be removing my gall bladder as my liver tumour was perilously close to it. I remember feeling really upset and sorry for my poor gall bladder, although I did not have a clue what it did. I was still furious with my bowel and liver for letting themselves get invaded by cancer, but I did not see what my poor gall bladder had done other than be unfortunate to have a less than careful neighbour. It appeared that Felix the Cat was going to attempt to take out a chunk of my liver and my gall bladder through keyhole surgery as well. (There are videos on YouTube showing this, but I still haven't plucked up the nerve to watch.)

I knew that the next big step was to let the children know. I had deliberately not told them of the liver tumour at the beginning as there had been no clear treatment plan at the time. I wanted to get the first success under my belt before tackling the next stage.

As soon as I got home, I had to figure out how to bring this up in conversation with Joseph and Lois. I decided to do it in a relaxed 'Oops, sorry, didn't I tell you?' way and tell them that I had a little spot of cancer in my liver which they really should take out, so I would be popping back into hospital a second time. They were not to worry, though, as the first op was fine, and this would be, too. I tried so hard to affect a tone of 'Oh yeah, this is just a routine bit of surgery', hardly worth mentioning, really! They were slightly worried about this, but, I thought at the time, not overly concerned. Time would tell …

The greatest glory in living lies not in never falling, but in rising every time we fall.

Nelson Mandela

CHAPTER EIGHT

❋

Another op ...

It was an early start on a brisk October morning. The only other time I remember getting up at this hour was on Christmas day when I was five years old. Same butterflies, but these were bad dudes – black gothic butterflies, not the frothy pink ones of childhood.

My mind was being unhelpful and filling my head with all sorts of unpleasant scenarios. I had always thought the bowel resection was a simpler operation, just a bit of plumbing that needed unblocking and rerouting. Whereas the liver, well, that was one serious piece of kit! In the hierarchy of my body, my mind in its blissful ignorance had organized it by importance, something like this (this is not my pronouncement on the severity of cancer, of course).

Organs I'm least happy to lose in order of importance:

1. Brain (can't live without)

2. Heart (ditto)

3. Lungs (can't last long without breathing)

4. Liver (serious stuff)

5. Stomach (can bypass it these days)

6. Kidneys (there's a spare)

7. Bowel (bit of plumbing, but like most plumbing, things go bad quickly if blocked)

8. Breasts (could do without if I had to)

9. Women's bits (still not sure what they do)

10. Other bits (ditto)

Bits I would accept losing:

1. Tonsils

2. Appendix

3. Ingrowing toenails

4. Teeth

➡

> **Bits I would be delighted to lose:**
>
> **1.** Double chin
>
> **2.** Bunions
>
> **3.** Varicose veins
>
> **4.** Birth marks and wrinkles

My partner drove me to the Churchill Hospital, while my mum and my dad stayed at home, looking after the children and trying to keep everything normal for them; after all, it was a regular school day.

As we drove along the M40 to Oxford, the radio piled on the anxiety by informing me that Steve Jobs had passed away from cancer that very night. A bad omen. I now felt even more nervous, especially as it was my first visit to this hospital. We parked and, speechless, we watched the occupant of the car parked next to us struggle out of his seat. For all the apples in the world, he was the spitting image of Steve Jobs. While we are on the subject of Steve Jobs: he had an industry-leading company, a massive brain, a compelling personal brand and enough black polo necks stashed away to last him until he was 100-years-old. If *he* had no leverage against cancer, what hope for the rest of us with our more mediocre bargaining chips?

As I was shown my room in the Upper GI Ward, I had the unfortunate shock of witnessing what appeared to be the wedding of the undead. A poor unfortunate soul was walking slowly up the ward with two enormous oxygen canisters pulled behind him on a trolley complete with clanking chains, accompanied by not one but two attendees both carrying a drain and bag of blood from goodness knows what orifice. The chains clanged loudly with every step he took. I expected to smell incense. My jaw fell open, and it took all my strength not to run for my life.

I was settled into my room in time to see my liver surgeon, Felix the Cat, doing his pre-op rounds and informing me that he was taking me down in an hour and that the operation would take three or four hours. As the liver is a huge dense organ made up of blood, the biggest risk when cutting into it was bleeding to death. So he explained there was a real chance I would end up in intensive care afterwards if they had trouble controlling the bleeding. He would remove as much of the liver as was necessary as well as the gall bladder for fear of the cancer spreading further, and I would wake up with a drain in my side, plus the usual paraphernalia. He intended to do the op by keyhole, but if there were any complications, he would, of course, slice me open like a fresh loaf of bread. Delicious. All said with a large smile on his face!

There is very little point in me trying to describe the level of pain from a liver resection as I have found that pain is the first thing in your memory to fade, and I did not keep notes at the time. And besides all that, morphine has a habit of somewhat knocking you out. I do, however, remember this being less painful than the bowel operation.

I stayed in hospital for six days and had various visitors, including my parents who, by now, were braving up to my partner and demanding their slot by my bedside. However, the visit with my children on day 3 was upsetting. I was in a lot of pain and suffering sickness. My morphine pump was not working, and the veins in my hands were shot to pieces. I pointed this out to the nurse, but she still insisted on giving me an antiemetic through my collapsed vein – the pain was excruciating. Finally, she realized, removed it and found another vein. Unfortunately, my son witnessed this, and has never wanted to visit me in hospital since.

My friend Jo and her husband Kim and daughter Lauren drove over the next day with my daughter. Lois had the look of someone who had just stepped off Nemesis at Alton Towers.

After much chat and inspecting of new tubes and wounds, we decided to shuffle down to the newsagent in the lobby and my jaw fell open ...

'WHSmith is looking for sadistic torturers to be in charge of book displays at leading cancer hospital, The Churchill.'

By the look of it, they had an enthusiastic response to their advertisement as the book display proudly promoted memoirs from people dying of cancer, memoirs of people abused as children, memoirs of people abusing their pets and memoirs of children dying. Not even a memoir from a celebrity chef or gardener among them, and they usually feature pretty high up on my torture list. Somebody must have thought long and hard about how the target audience in this specialist cancer hospital would like to spend their days and decided, 'Let's see what these hard nuts are really made of!'

Food was also not their forte, so my partner brought in freshly made soup as I could not tolerate what passes for food in an NHS ward. I don't want you to get the wrong idea about this hospital, though: the surgeons are excellent, patients can use the piano in the café and there is a wig shop.

My surgery was successful, and my pathology results were good, with clear margins. Felix the Cat this time affected an air of general disinterest and underplayed most things to the point that I almost felt he thought I had Munchausen's syndrome. He was also followed around by at least 12 other doctors or disciples, and I guess it helped convince me that he could do miracles.

The nursing, however, was less successful, and on my first night after surgery, I called for over an hour for assistance. Eventually, a nurse turned up and said that if I had trouble reaching anyone again, to please pick up my water jug and throw it at the door! Excellent advice, but not one I decided to add to my list. Needless to say, my brother got to hear about this and turned up armed with a list of questions and demands from the staff. We all know better than to try and fob off my brother when his eyebrows attach themselves to the top of his head and he adopts a look on his face as if he is licking a nettle. Run for your lives! Or start speaking fast!

List of facts about liver resections

1. Treating liver metastases with surgery is becoming more normal – it is the gold standard of treatment options.

2. As the liver can regenerate, surgeons can remove up to 75 per cent of the liver nowadays. The liver can regrow in as little as three months.

3. The liver is the most common area that bowel cancer can spread to because the venous drainage of the colon is through the portal vein that drains into the liver.

4. Liver resections used to be high-risk operations as previously about a fifth of patients died from haemorrhaging. ➡

5. Sometimes there is an option to remove liver metastases before the primary tumour as secondary tumours are considered faster-growing.

6. In general, surgeons consider liver resections if there are less than five lesions and two segments of the liver (you have four lobes divided into eight segments) are clear. However, there are now more and more surgical techniques such as RFA (radio frequency ablation) to treat those lesions or segments that surgery cannot reach.

* * *

Since I was diagnosed, and while waiting the six weeks for chemo to start after my liver operation, I had plenty of time to muse about my disease and to contemplate most of the cancer *faux pas* in existence. From reading the endless blogs and forum discussions on the subject on the Internet, there is no doubt that whether you are the one with cancer or the one looking in, you will have a shared awkwardness in common. So this is my attempt to try and navigate a way through.

For some reason, a language attaches itself to cancer that no other illness suffers from. With one in three of us facing cancer at some point in our lives, I guess it is a fascination most of us will flirt with, and while the intent is often good, fear or awkwardness leads everyone to fall into the cliché trap sooner or later.

As you know, I would never want anyone to feel awkward, and so, in addition to listing the main *faux pas*, I have also tried to suggest alternatives. But, ultimately, as with anything, it is the way you say it and what is really in your heart.

List of cancer faux pas

1. *Stay positive.*

2. *You will fight this.*

3. I know *you will be okay.*

4. *Cancer picked the wrong person to have a fight with.*

5. *If anyone can beat cancer, then you can!*

6. *I know someone who has/had cancer of the* (insert any cancer other than yours) *and is fine now.*

7. *My friend/aunt/mum had cancer, went downhill very quickly and died in agony.*

8. *You must try the xyz cure: so and so had two months to live, ate a mushroom and is fine now.*

9. *But you don't look ill/But you look good!*

10. *None of us knows when we are going to die. You could get knocked down by a bus tomorrow.*

11. *We are all only sent what we can handle/What doesn't kill you makes you stronger.*

Bear in mind that most cancer patients will have heard the 'positive' statement hundreds of times, and after the one-hundredth-and-one time, it will begin to sound like an accusation or, worse still, a demand. It can also feel like an attempt to 'shut down' any further discussion for fear of sounding anything other than continually upbeat.

One of my only excuses for being rude is when someone tries to tell me a ghastly tale of death without first checking on my current well-being. This is chronically insensitive, and I can think of no other example where this type of conversational tactic is used. I now ask as soon as the words 'I know someone ...' is out of the person's mouth, 'Excuse me, does this story end well? If not, I don't want to hear it please.' Nine times out of ten people open and shut their mouths wordlessly and then shut up for good.

When you are growing your own peculiar brand of cancer, you will feel endlessly intrigued by it and initially will search out other cases of people with *your* type of cancer in the search for knowledge. Of course, there are many commonalities between cancers, and we can all learn a lot from each other, but when talking to someone about the success of the x or y treatment, bear in mind that this will not be terribly useful to someone who does not share your cancer type or your prognosis. While this story will do wonders for your spirit if it ends well, be careful to keep it relevant. And go gently on the advice.

The question of looks is a thorny one. Cancer plays havoc with your looks and self-confidence, and so it is always lovely to hear a genuine compliment about how well you look. I only objected when I felt it was said with a little suspicion, a sort of 'Are you sure you are that ill because you don't look it?' Here are my alternative suggestions.

List of helpful things to say to cancer patients

1. *Gosh, I did not expect you to look that good, but how are you really feeling?*

I always felt such a relief when someone softened this with a genuine 'How are you *really* feeling?' It stopped me feeling ungrateful for a genuine compliment. It also meant that I did not feel the need to follow up with a curt 'Cheers, but I feel crap!'

2. *Please say if we should go now to give you some rest/ Shall we limit our visiting for a bit to allow you some time to recover properly without needing to talk to us?*

I would rather drop dead with exhaustion than ask someone to leave, but there were many occasions when my body was screaming out to lie down. Once someone picked up on this and was sensitive to my new limitations, I was able to be honest about how I felt.

3. *Can I pick up anything for you as I am popping to the shops?*

How do you respond to that? It is open-ended and makes us feel awkward for asking as we never know if we are sending you out of your way. But if you get into the habit of being specific about where you are going and ask if you can pick up something from the pharmacy or drop off a child, for example, it will be

→

incredibly helpful. You might want to be even braver and just say, 'I'm coming round in an hour to mow your lawn/put the washing on/cook you a meal.' Heaven!

4. *It must be a real pain to miss coming out with the girls/I imagine you must get fed up of being exhausted and/or in pain all the time.*

When I was really ill, all I wanted was for people to understand how I felt and to be heard. Having someone really listen and then play those fears, disappointments or that sadness back to you is a great relief.

5. *I miss going out to lunch together/I miss you at work.*

This is so important to hear. So much has changed, and it is good to have this acknowledged and to be able to feel you are really missed and not forgotten.

6. *Please don't feel bad if you have to cancel at the last minute. Just play it by ear, I'll understand.*

I still feel bad about cancelling plans, but it is a relief to hear this as it takes off masses of pressure. I no longer feel I need to force myself to go out or make promises if I am uncertain how I will feel.

7. *Would you like me to tell you what the gossip is about (insert the name of your boss here)/Shall I tell you what I got up to over the weekend?*

➡

Not 'arf! Unfortunately, some people feel guilty about telling me some of the fab things they have been up to or bits of juicy gossip in case it makes me feel bad as I cannot do the same. I loved it and it took me out of myself for a moment.

8. *Chin up, lass, one day at a time!*

This is infinitely more pleasing than to be told to be positive! I am not suggesting I wanted to waterboard anyone who kept telling me to be positive, but I did feel twinges of annoyance – the sort of feeling you get from people who keep trying to get you to dance at parties or weddings.

9. *I hope you're as well as possible.*

It takes the sting out of everything and shows real compassion for that person.

The Swiss-American psychiatrist Elisabeth Kübler-Ross wrote knowledgeably about the five stages of dealing with personal trauma. It is called the grief curve, and it is said that anyone facing big-scale upset will go through the following stages:

Denial: Yep, got that one, and to be honest, there is nothing wrong with a bit of denial to help you gradually come to terms with things. It is a basic defence mechanism as our mind instinctively tries to protect us. This is okay as a short-term respite, until the new reality filters in.

Anger: I was angry with myself for delaying visits to the doctor and angry with my doctor for sending me away twice. It was not really a rage, just a gentle sort of annoyance. Maybe in my case, I am still waiting for real anger!

Bargaining: See below.

Depression: This can often manifest itself as a practice run or a dress rehearsal for what might happen to the family if I died. Chemo depression is another thing altogether and can naturally occur at each cycle.

Acceptance: The point when you find some kind of emotional detachment from what may happen to you. You often reach it before your family does who will also need to go through their own five stages of grief.

I would also add a new stage:

Guilt: I felt a real sense of being responsible for ruining everyone's lives.

With regard to denial, I did not have much time for that. And, to repeat, I never really suffered much from anger. But bargaining, that's definitely the one for me! I'd willingly give up organs, vanity and control over my future, I'd accept loss of sex drive and some pain and sickness, but I'd bargain all the way to hang on to humour, occasional rebellion, wine and – life!

I figured I have had an interesting and full life and tempted the arrival of the Grim Reaper a number of times, so it is a waste of time complaining and regretting anything. And one thing's for certain, there's nothing like the Sly Old Fox to knock the shine off your mojo!

You could have planted Mr (or Dr as he obviously would be called) Darcy scrubbed up in his hospital blues and asked him to take my pulse with his long sensual fingers ... and even he would not have noticed the slightest quickening. Many things get chucked into the lost-property basket as you go along: bits of body parts, bikinis, hipster trousers, short-term memory ... But one thing I hope has not gone missing, or at least will be returned to me at the end of term, is my sense of humour and optimism.

As I was about to now enter phase 3, the chemo long slog, this was to become more important than ever.

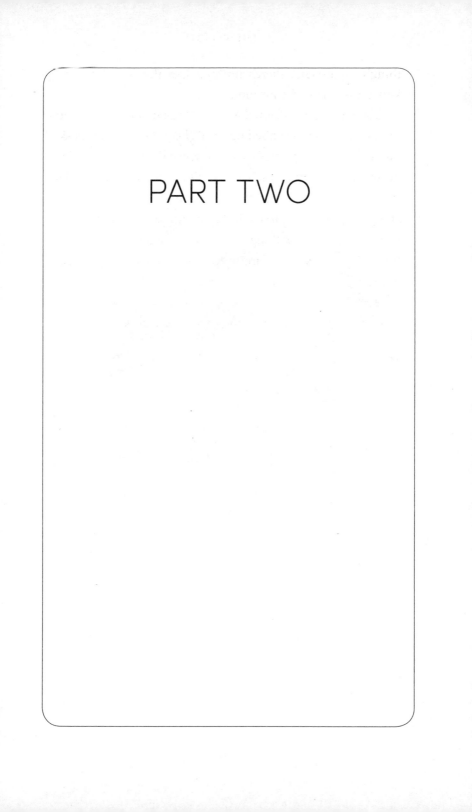

PART TWO

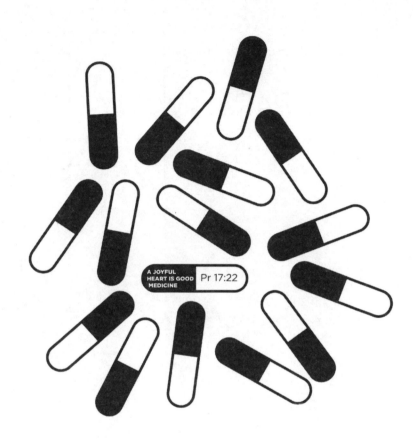

A JOYFUL HEART IS GOOD MEDICINE

Pr 17:22

CHAPTER NINE

*

Chemo time

Give me my surgeon's sharp claws over chemo anytime please … I hated chemo with a vengeance, so this next part deals with my biggest challenge. When I was able, I kept a blog of some of my experiences over at www.bananagiraffes.com. It was a deliberate attempt to inject some nonsense and to distract me from the anticipated side effects as well as keeping my friends and family informed. I had no idea how tired I would become – or how successful the blog would become. I had around 50,000 hits the first year just through word of mouth, and got to meet and make some new and now close friends. This was my very first entry:

Chemo eve, am I being naive?

I hope I don't revisit this, my very first blog post, and marvel at my optimism for not letting chemo dominate my life over the next six months!

Since having been diagnosed with secondary bowel cancer in August 2011, I have been swept along by the medical profession from one consultation to another. From one major operation to another. And now, finally, I have breathing space before chemo starts next week. So while I am still deluded into thinking that I can do this, I am setting up my blog to distract me and hopefully give hope to anyone else going through a similar experience.

People wiser than me tell me that positivity and meditation will get me through unscathed mentally and physically. So I am drawn to using this 'sabbatical' to do things I would never consider in a million years getting around to.

I don't know what I will want to do when I complete my treatment and am fighting fit again, but I do know that I am now officially sick of daytime TV … they just don't cater for vegetating chemo patients with a limited stay-awake time.

So I am looking for your help. I need challenges, things to set my mind to and focus me anywhere but the Jeremy Kyle Show.

The challenge can be as obscure, oblique or just plain silly as you like – in fact, the crazier, the better!

The challenges poured in quickly, and as I know I have a great skill in prevarication, I decided I would publish them in a feeble attempt to stop me ducking everyone.

List of challenges

1. Play Christmas carols at the Churchill Hospital dressed as a banana giraffe. *Done.*

2. Do some Banksy-style street art.

3. Edit a science blog on cancer. *Done.*

4. Brew my own beer using bananas.

5. Build a 40ft Banana Giraffe sticking out the roof of my house (see Shark in Oxford for inspiration). *Half done.*

6. Be interviewed speaking in a posh voice on live radio. *Done.*

7. Build an angry Banana Giraffes app.

8. Persuade Sheikh Mohammed Bin Rashid Al Maktoum that horses and camels are *sooo* 2011 and that his next investment should be in banana giraffe racing.

9. Enter a banana giraffes swimathon team for charity (maybe not the channel yet?).

10. Organize a banana giraffes flash mob.

11. Organize a banana giraffes fun run or race for life. *Done.*

12. Appear on various TV shows to raise money for bowel cancer charities.

13. Write my own book on getting through cancer. *Done.*

Oh dear, looking through this list as I finish chemo, I realize that I only managed five and a half challenges! I am blaming naivety – and am extending the end date of these challenges indefinitely.

* * *

One of the many unjust things about the health system is the difference in level of care and equipment between the private and NHS hospitals. But as I was being treated courtesy of BUPA, I had been offered the opportunity to have a porta-cath inserted in my chest which would be sealed in and used to take in the chemo, rather than the more painful option of having the chemo pumped into a vein in my hand each time, or having a PICC line inserted. The portacath – a tiny medical appliance inserted under the skin – was a mixed blessing for me, and I was not yet ready to call it my friend. But as it was rather scarily plugged into my jugular, I had to treat it with some respect. It was like an alien life force, and when I lay down, it swelled up, highlighting the tubes in my chest.

Every time a surgeon went through the consent form and read the list of things that could go wrong, I had an irrepress-ible urge to laugh. This minor operation was no different, as my Kiwi surgeon told me laconically that he could puncture my lungs when putting in the portacath (or USB port as my brother calls it). If this happened, he would simply stick a tube in and blow them up again! Oh, what a relief because, for a moment, I was nervous … I should have given him an animal name, but I was struggling with laconic Kiwi animals, so I broke out of the zoo for a moment and called him Dirty Harry as that was the closest analogy I could find.

Unfortunately, you are only sedated during this procedure,

so to take my mind off this possibility and the rummaging around Dirty Harry was doing in my chest, he told me to think of something nice for the next hour.

The 'minor' operation left me feeling really rotten. My chest felt awful and the pain rippled continuously across my neck and back. I had no idea why, but from reading posts on forums, this can sometimes happen when putting in a porta-cath. Presumably the nerves had been severely interfered with as it took over three weeks to settle down.

After the operation, I was told to go home and sleep it off. No one told my Tibetan terrier, Luca, who clearly had other ideas.

How do you tell a dog off who has taken it upon himself to be the house alarm clock? My daughter Lois is usually up before 7am to catch her school bus at 7.30am. So imagine Luca's dilemma when the house was still asleep at 7.30am that Sat-urday morning. Determined to come to the rescue, he leapt off my bed and shot into Lois's room and, resting both his front legs on her pillow, howled into her ear. When she did not immediately respond, he jumped onto her bed and swiped her with his paws (or pandys as we like to call them).

By which time the whole house was awake, including my teenage son. And, of course, in true dog style, Luca went straight back to sleep. And I am told that dogs are natural healers …

* * *

Now for the hardcore bit – my first experience of chemo.

My best friend Jenny decided she was going to take me to my very first chemo session in her open-top sports car. At least we were going to start this in style! The chemo room was full to overflowing with people wired up to machines that sounded eerily like a field of crickets clicking away. But it appeared to be a popular place to hang out as there were no seats available, and so I was put in an upright uncomfortable seat by the radiator and told that was all they had that day as there were too many patients and not enough staff. So far, not so good.

Then, in a voice that could be heard two floors down, my chemo nurse said, 'Oh, you have a portacath, that's only for patients who are private!' Smashing. 'But it makes no difference, you all get the same treatment here, love.' Ouch, why did the floor not swallow me up? 'Hopefully, we can empty these seats in the next hour', she continued, pointing to reclining seats full of human beings who looked shocked and guilty. I am not having a go at the nurses who were wonderful, but at the wretched system that plays with people's lives when they are at their lowest ebb. Complaining about someone about to inject you with toxic material makes the risk of complaining about your food in a restaurant child's play! I zipped up my mouth, like the rest of the patients, and obediently sat there, waiting to be nuked.

One ECG and X-ray later to check why I was still in pain from the so-called luxury port, I was finally wired up to go. Luckily, I was extravagantly distracted by Jenny, who came equipped with a bag of treats and a lubricated jaw until the drip of chemo finally spat out its last mouthful two hours later.

Unfortunately, a woman in the next room had a severe reaction to Oxaliplatin, and I witnessed the horrible choking sounds and panic as her throat went into spasms. The nurses drew the curtain around her, applied a hot beanbag to her throat and tried to calm her down. After an age, they re-emerged and glanced over guiltily in my direction, hoping (mistakenly) I had been rendered temporarily blind and deaf.

Apart from red ants running down my back and into my pants from the steroids, an unnerving experience of my throat closing up and painful tingling in my jaw when I tried to eat, I did not have too many bad side effects during the infusion. To avoid the dreaded sickness, though, I had to take another dose of steroids at 5pm that kept me bouncing off the walls all night.

I realize now that the operations were somehow easier to deal with. There was a beginning and an end to them. I would feel crap for four to six weeks, but in reducing levels. In contrast, chemo cranked up the feeling of crapness as you went through. There was no way of predicting how you would feel after each session, and there was no rhythm to it. For example, I felt relieved on Wednesday and Thursday, but dreadful on Friday and Saturday. The tiredness was nothing like I can describe properly: it was not a sleepy tiredness but a 'leg and arm twitching, can't concentrate' tiredness. I promise I will *never* complain of ordinary tiredness again! And all I seemed to want to eat were sharp, salty flavours to take the edge off the sickness. Even then, everything tasted of cardboard. You need to get into the right frame of mind before chemo, but there are a few practical things you can buy or suggest to your supporters beforehand.

List of things to buy or do before chemo starts

1. A new luxury pillow.
   (My dad bought me this and my mum bought some new bedding – it felt delicious.)

2. A new V-shaped cushion to make it easy for you to sit up in bed to read.

3. Downloading some favourite music onto your MP3.

4. Box sets of your favourite programmes, preferably comedy or something distracting but not taxing.

5. Luxury bath treats, ideally organic, and magnesium bath salts, or Epsom salts, to help with aches and pain.

6. Tempting snacks to nibble on to help with nausea.

7. Chewing gum to get rid of the chemo taste in your mouth.

8. Earmuffs, scarves, gloves, thick socks and slippers, if on chemo drugs such as Oxaliplatin which affect the nerve endings in hands, feet and throat.

9. A pair of thin gloves so you can get stuff out of the fridge, but still feel them.

10. Getting any essential dental work done beforehand as this is not recommended during chemo.
    (This may not always be possible depending on

➡

the operation and treatment schedule suggested
by your surgeon.)

11. Getting eyebrows tattooed if your chemo is a
hair-loss type regime.
(Mine was not.)

12. Exploring whether you have a local salon that
supplies and cuts wigs, preferably made from
human hair if you can afford it.

13. Asking your oncologist to prescribe a light
sleeping pill.
(A good night's sleep without sickness works
wonders with cancer.)

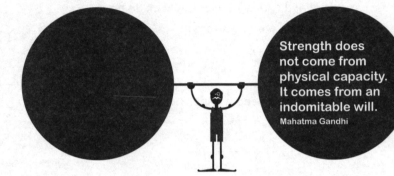

Strength does not come from physical capacity. It comes from an indomitable will.
Mahatma Gandhi

✳

CHAPTER TEN

Coping with chemo depression

One thing your medical team doesn't tell you much about is the chemo depression that creeps up on you until you think you have always been like this. It is only after the fog lifts that you remember this is not the norm. I struggled with it throughout the eight months I was on chemo, but I was so lucky to have the most supportive and unselfish family around me at all times.

If love and kindness alone could be prescribed for recovery, I would have been cured on the very first day of chemo. In an attempt to lift me out of my sinking mood, my amazing brother and his girlfriend Lucie turned up for a Sunday family dinner with armfuls of beautifully wrapped original artworks. They had handpicked a number of quotes to lift my spirits, and David, who is a creative designer, had illustrated them all and framed them as a set. Simply looking at them gave me incredible strength.

* * *

Keeping up my spirits was tricky. If I could have had a pound for every time someone told me to stay positive, I would be in Barbados right now. If, of course, I could get my colostomy bag past Customs and Excise!

Never did I need more reminding of this simple but true saying as I did after the side effects kicked in from my first chemo.

I felt dog rough, so I eventually gave in and headed back to hospital to alert the chemo nurses to my worsening symptoms: night sweats, achy bones and skin, tingling fingers, sickness, diarrhoea and the sort of wipe-out exhaustion that does not let you sleep. This was all met with a reassuring 'Ah yes, this is normal, you are having a reaction to the chemo drugs', and advice to stop the tablets for a few days and to rest as much as possible.

My friend Alison decided I needed to keep my focus and contacted Radio Cherwell, the hospital radio station, to arrange a radio interview with me as a precursor to the playing of Christmas songs dressed as a banana giraffe at the Churchill Hospital. This was followed quickly by a series of interviews with Malcolm Boyden from BBC Oxford. That shocked me out of my downward spiral. I like the adrenaline of live radio. I am much better on radio than on TV where my nerves get picked up and I either talk r-e-a-l-l-y s-l-o-w-l-y or gabble and twitch. But I was surprised as everyone where my 'posh' voice came from. My upbeat message obviously connected with some of the listeners as I had comments on my blog later that day as well as people turning up to my Christmas banana giraffe concert!

* * *

Meanwhile, I adjusted my expectations and learnt to grab that half hour in the day when I was capable of doing what I used to do before the cancer struck. It was wonderful to feel human.

But all good things have to come to an end (why?), and after a few days I tried again with the Capecitabine tablets. They are not for the faint-hearted, and I was dreading having to take them again. It had only been a short while, but I was already on less than good terms with chemo and knew what I was facing. So, as I prepared to reintroduce chemo into my body, I wrote the following list:

Checklist to reintroduce chemo after a break

1. *Check.* All cranial cavities filled with a spray can of polystyrene foam.

2. *Check.* Two litres of sand inserted under entire layer of skin.

3. *Check.* Hormone 'balance' adjusted to menopausal harridan levels.

4. *Check.* Portacath ready with imported virus to shut down mainframe activity before it can be completed.

5. *Check.* Network connection disconnected.

6. *Final check.* Sleep levels adjusted to Margaret Thatcher 'running a country' level (apologies to anyone reading this younger than 35, but, for reference, four hours).

Thank you, doc, I think that all seems reasonable. We are good to go again.

I was determined to get my head around this chemo challenge better the next time, but was pondering why my body had not managed to fight off the enemy-invading forces. I eventually came to the conclusion that my white blood cells after an early fight had decided to sign an armistice with the enemy army.

My nutritionist informed me that although I had a healthy number of white blood cells, the little chaps they call the NK or killer squad were not active enough. They had allowed the cancer cells to set up base in France (or my bowel), and if that were not enough of a liberty, they had let them go unchallenged into my liver (luckily, for historical comparisons, not England!).

So, what was the plan to turn this sleeping NK squad into the feared Foreign Legion or, probably more appropriately, the current British army?

Well, I had two plans – Plan A and Plan B. Plan A was the conventional 'operations and chemo' package. My medical team had advised me to embrace chemo rather than to see it as the enemy for mind and body. Plan B was my back-up plan. As my nutritionist explained, we had to eradicate the terrain that allowed these conditions to flourish in the first case. Needless to say, it involved taking enough tablets and drinks a day to induce a gag reflex.

Meanwhile, my dad, who had been the driving force behind Plan B and had spent more hours in research than Alexander Fleming, had brought a small pharmacy to my house and did spot audit checks to calculate if I was taking all the drugs.

I should point out here for relevance that my dad is a retired accountant, although we all know you can never retire that part of your brain. Anyway, he then came up with an even more audacious plan. He had found a new product that was so well respected it cost more than a small flat in Great

Missenden to buy (we are talking post HS2 train link here, so I am not exaggerating too wildly!). However, it appeared that you could obtain this product at a fraction of the cost from a pharmacy in Budapest.

So my dad, who can do sums in his head so fast it would give my brain whiplash, calculated if he could earn enough air miles to fly to Budapest and buy the product from the chemist's, we'd be quids in. The answer was yes!

I don't know what else to say other than my dad is my superhero.

This is how the conversation went: 'Let me get this straight, you are going to fly to Budapest on the 8.30am flight, meet a women you have just made contact with through a friend in Israel, hand over money for a suitcase of medicine and get on the next flight back home without leaving the airport? And you don't think any of this will alarm the authorities at the airport?' 'No, why should it?' said Superdad, adjusting his flat cap nervously.

It did seem too good to be true, but these were the actual events that unfolded in Budapest. Here is the background. My dad had researched a product called Avemar and had set about securing a six-month supply in the most economical way possible. Having found out that the product was manufactured and sold in Hungary, my dad dusted down his little black book and remembered that, on a visit to Israel, he had got talking to a lovely lady called Eva, who had lived in Budapest during the war. Her story was worthy of a film script. For much of the war, she had been hiding in a mine shaft until she was discovered and imprisoned. Thankfully, she survived and emigrated to Israel. In passing, she must have mentioned that she had a niece in Budapest called Erika, and my dad had tucked this away for future reference.

Erika is a woman who, in the truest Jewish sense, takes hospitality as an Olympic sport: not only did she research where the product could be purchased even cheaper, but she sourced it and made the two-hour journey to the airport to save my dad the time and bother. And if that was not enough, she came armed with Hungarian wine and chocolates for my mother and me.

* * *

Anyway, I have tantalized you long enough about Plan B. Please note: *This is my own personal protocol based on my circumstances and blood results. It is advisable to get your own, but I thought this has such useful information that I would share it with you in the next chapter, 'Brain Food'.*

One of the many things I learnt to ask for during cancer treatment was a copy of my files and blood tests. As I have no medical training, I had to learn to interpret these carefully, and my medical team can testify to many an anxious conversation, where I misinterpreted all manner of things. It is useful to keep copies for two reasons:

1. Records, files and appointments can get mixed up or go missing. It does not hurt to keep your own, and for those of you born before 1970 when it was considered the height of rudeness to question anyone in authority, this is quite normal!

2. If you decide to help your immune system along a bit and see a nutritionist, it helps to have records of your latest blood results so that he or she can tailor your treatment accordingly.

* * *

It takes time to cope with the ups and downs that accompany chemotherapy. This is quite normal, but each cycle I completely forgot it and suffered from chemo depression during the first week of treatment. It completely altered my perception of most things, and tears were a frequent side effect. One unexpected target for my latest set of tears was my car.

I am not saying our village is boring, but Pamela, my dear old seven-seater Mercedes, was the most popular attraction in the village for a while. At one stage, I can recall having nearly all of Year 5 in the back of her on one journey home from school. And most of these in the two seats facing backward.

I started to feel better as the second week approached, but my mind was still not my own yet and I was still liable to cry at the slightest thing. Maybe I was being a bit too emotional about a tin box, but you know the way the sun can shine with such intensity to make even the most mundane objects glow with such mystical qualities that you cannot take your eyes off them? Well, Pamela for about four years (while the children were at Little Kingshill Primary School) had that special light shine on her most of the time.

It may, of course, have been this, or it may have been the fact that nothing else passes for entertainment in our village. A bit like Clement Freud's impression when asked to comment on New Zealand: 'I find it hard to say, because when I was there, it appeared to be shut.'

But whatever it was, she was a 1¼-ton treasure (and yes, my children did ask my dad to convert this to kilograms which he did in nanoseconds), sadly packed off to be crushed, still thick with childhood memories. Many tears were shed.

Meanwhile, my son tried his best to come up with other attractions in our house to encourage in the village. Thankfully, not the 'sick mother' attraction but plenty of mock rifle ranges in our not so peaceful garden. In stark contrast, my daughter's answer was, and still is, to bake. Not one person left our house without a homemade cake or biscuit to comfort them. Many charities have benefited from her awesome fund-raising talents, with 'giraffe-shaped, rain-soaked biscuits' being just one of them!

Jenny presented me with my very first challenge a few days after I had been diagnosed. Knowing that Lois and I would donate a kidney for the chance of seeing the Spanish Riding School, she had booked a couple of tickets for their first London tour in five years. I remember thinking it was a daunting three months in the future, and I could not be sure how I would be feeling or whether my mum, who has hippo-phobia, would have to go in my place. (Hippophobia is a fear of horses. It is totally unfair of me to have a laugh about it as my mum had to conquer her fear after taking on my horsey duties and accompanying Lois to the stables. No mean feat when Welly, the pony, was less than gentlemanly and liable to put the willies up anyone ...) Thankfully, for both of us, that was not the case.

So, after banking a load of sleep and taking an industrial supply of hand wipes and a promise to wear my Michael Jackson mask as my white blood count was still very low, I set off with Lois, determined to avoid the great unwashed.

It worked a treat as, miraculously, we appeared to re-enact the parting of the Red Sea wherever we went. We were warned that the horses were easily spooked and no flash photography was allowed, which, like all good citizens, we ignored. I figured if the horses could put up with red flashes going off around the arena, my terrorist mask was the least of their problems.

The grace of the horses and riders brought a lump to my throat, and once they filled the arena with the regal sound of

Handel's *Water Music Suite No. 1 in F Major: Overture*, I was openly weeping, but I would not have missed it for the world. These treats really lifted my spirits, and any discomfort was well worth the pain.

As you undoubtedly have already concluded, I am a little bit spoilt, and yes, Superdad and Supermum were waiting outside to drive us back home. This happily coincided with a rush to Wembley for *The X Factor* quarterfinal results, so traffic was beginning to resemble a Beijing Expressway. Never one to sit in a traffic jam when there is an illegal bus route he can take, my dad set off on a mission to beat the traffic. We thought we had got away with it until a ticket arrived in the post a week later. Poor Dad!

* * *

The thing about chemo is this: you need the promise of treats to get you through the days when all you want to do is sleep and wake up in six months' time. But some treats are never as good as you had led yourself to believe. Take baths, for example. You long for a bath at the end of the day to ease aches, warm up your skin and let your mind float away. So how come that within seconds of easing yourself in, you feel hot and bothered with an urgent need to escape? But you cannot because you poured a pint of magnesium salts into your bath as your nutritionist had told you it helps you sleep and is absorbed through your skin. So you sit clutching your knees until you feel you have got your money's worth, get out and can flop into your bed. The same can be said for cakes or savoury treats. I sent my mother loopy behaving like a modern-day Henry VIII on steroids, demanding new daily flavours and foods to help with the chemo sickness: 'This week

I fancy macaroons, but only the ones with dark chocolate on that you get in that shop way yonder (the next county)' ... only to put them to my lips, taste the now familiar flavour of cardboard box and vow never to eat them again.

My dad, of course, took this as a fabulous opportunity to add even more ginger to my daily juices, assuming I would not be able to taste or complain about it. Sadly for him, ginger is one of the flavours that get a free chemo pass, and so I was very vocal in my distaste for this, too, despite his good-humoured 'It's good for you'. Everything my dad gives me is 'good for me' I have since found, thus halting any feeble attempts to refuse it.

List of ideal treats while on chemo

1. Going to the cinema in the afternoon when there are not many people or germs about.

2. Attending a daytime art or photography course if you can find one flexible enough to book *ad hoc* when you feel up to it.

3. Getting out for a coffee or cake once a week.

4. A spot of online shopping so you can look forward to a nice treat arriving in the post.

5. I tried to book at last one trip or treat in the calendar every session to focus on.

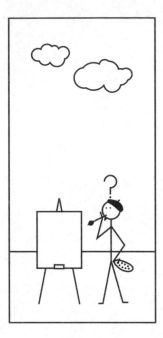

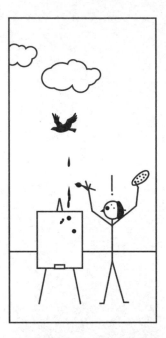

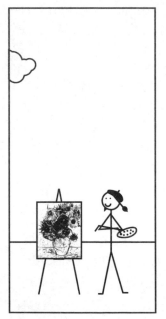

The art of life is to turn even unpleasant things to advantage.

BETTY REEKIE

✳

Brain food

In a nutshell (a large one!), the following is my protocol based on information from my nutritionist. I have removed the specific dosages and timings as each person is different, but I hope it will prompt some discussion and thoughts. All in-formation has been provided courtesy of my nutritionist Juliet Haywood.

My nutritional profile

Centaurium by Bioforce: helps reduce acid reflux by strengthening the sphincter around the opening to the stomach.

Asafoetida Plus by Pukka: helpful for reducing painful wind.

Biobran sachet (1000mg) by The Really Healthy Company: helps boost immunity by activating Natural Killer cells, T-lymphocytes, B-lymphocytes and dendritic

➡

cells. Natural Killer cells seek out malignant cells to annihilate them. They naturally migrate to rapidly dividing cells. Dendritic cells gather up pathogenic cells and present them to the NK cells. Cancer cells can emit substances that suppress the maturation of the dendritic cells, leading to tumour tolerance. Biobran is able to help the dendritic cells withstand this and reach maturity so they can work more effectively with the NK cells. Biobran also helps boost interleukin 2, a substance produced by the immune cells to help mount a defence against viruses, bacteria and malignant cells. It also helps reduce inflammation. In addition, Biobran can help safeguard against some of the side effects of platinum-based chemotherapy drugs (any chemo drugs ending in 'platin' such as Oxaliplatin).

Acerola-C (500mg) by Nature's Plus: a Vitamin C, helpful for reducing your susceptibility to viruses.

Butyric Acid by Biocare: helps induce cell death in malignant cells within the colon and protect healthy colon cells.

Lipozyme by Biocare: an enzyme that breaks down fats. Lipozyme can help compensate if you no longer have a gall bladder.

Geo by New Vistas: developed to protect you from geopathic stress.

Liv 52 by Vedic: useful for liver detoxification and supporting liver function. It may help reduce raised liver

➡

enzymes. (You need to reduce this product once you are on chemotherapy.)

Yarrow by Herba Naturelle: has astringent qualities and can help reduce internal bleeding.

Caricol by Nutri Ltd: can help improve bowel movements in a gentle way.

Ashwagandha by Nutrition Herbs: helpful for adrenal support and improving your ability to withstand stress.

Nature's Biotics by Kiki: helps reduce gut fermentation and boost bowel flora. Cancer cells are fuelled by fermentation as they do not burn oxygen for energy like healthy cells. Good bowel flora helps police the gut and safeguard the body from absorbing pollutants that you have ingested. It can also help boost immune cells, synthesize certain nutrients and short-chain fatty acids.

Truefood Selenium 200Ug by Higher Nature: helps boost white blood cells called neutrophils. It reduces inflammation and boosts an important antioxidant called glutathione. Selenium helps boost T- and B-lymphocyte proliferation. It also helps increase NK cell levels; it bolsters interleukin 2 (an immune substance that helps fight malignant cells) and up-regulates cell-mediated immunity (immunity that comes from within the cell) and humoral immunity (immunity that comes from outside the cell).

Slippery Elm Powder by Baldwins: mix half a teaspoon in tepid water to form a paste and then add hot water

➡

to make a tea. This is helpful for reducing inflammation and pain throughout the whole of the GI tract.

Bio D Mulsion Forte by Biotics Research: helpful to boost cell differentiation and reduce cell proliferation.

VegEpa by Igennus (fish oils): helps reduce inflammation and induce cell apoptosis (death of old or malignant cells).

B12 Active by Enzymatic Therapy: helps reduce nerve tingling by enhancing nerve repair. It also helps boost the red blood cell count.

Glutamine Powder by Lamberts: helpful to strengthen and repair the gut wall. It is particularly helpful for those who have undergone bowel surgery. All lymphocytes are dependent on glutamine. Glutamine enhances their proliferation and stimulates cytokine release. Cytokines are the 'weapons' of the immune system. *In vitro* glutamine boosts both interleukin 2 and gamma interferon, two important cytokines.

Serraenzyme 80,000iu by Good Healthy Naturally: a powerful antiinflammatory.

One hour before retiring
Asphalia for Natural Sleep by Coghill Labs (optional): helps enhance sleep and boost melatonin. Melatonin is an important antioxidant that also boosts the cytokine interleukin 2. This immune substance has an important role in protecting you against pathogens. This could also be helpful in protecting against geopathic stress.

➡

Zinc Picolinate by Solgar: all T-lymphocytes (immune cells) are dependent on zinc. Zinc fires up Natural Killer cells that police the body killing pathogens and malignant cells. It also boosts circulating lymphocytes by increasing the production of thymulin, which enhances lymphocyte replication. It also helps increase neutrophils.

Nausea

Ginger Honey Tonic by New Chapter: take 1–2 teaspoons whenever you need it. It is helpful for nausea, and is anti-inflammatory and rich in antioxidants.

Foods

Green tea: drink 2–3 cups a day, ideally in the first part of the day and not with any food. This can help reduce NF Kappa B, an inflammatory protein. NF Kappa B can be instrumental in helping cancer cells migrate to other parts of the body.

Turmeric: Use this spice copiously in cooking. Cook in coconut oil with black pepper. This is a powerful antioxidant and can be helpful to reduce NF Kappa B. Avoid using a microwave oven as this can suppress immunity.

Mucilaginous foods: important to limit discomfort and pain in the bowel. Try eating one of the mucilaginous foods such as flax seeds or slippery elm, marshmallow root or aloe every day. Check with your doctor or a nutritionist.

* * *

I used to think Monday was an awful waste of a seventh of the week and would have been much happier with two Thursdays or two Fridays instead. But I must say that being unable to work through chemotherapy helped change my mind.

Admittedly, our local delicious tapas bar did help sugar the pill. You could often find me there on Mondays with either local friend Jo or non-local friend Alison, both ready to galvanize me into action if they rightly detected a note of indolence about me.

The one thing I was not expecting was how much chemo makes you ravenous, while, at the same time, making you nauseous. If I was not seated and eating by 12 noon, I was in danger of eating my young. Our friendly tapas bar learnt to collaborate with this indecently early arrival, and any shock they felt at being caught in their pyjamas was hurriedly hidden under a welcoming smile.

But I have to confess I sometimes did overdo things. I had taken to this positive mind-and-body thing so enthusiastically that I literally convinced myself that I was as fit and well as the next man (unless, of course, the next man was Jack Lemmon in *The Odd Couple*). My memory had also colluded in this farce and downplayed any knowledge of past surgeries or chemo drips. In fact, my old surgery sites (bowel and liver) took on the air of ancient elder statesmen who would scoff at the little chemo upstart and tell him in their day they practically let the surgeon rip me open while on nothing more than a swig of whisky.

This is obviously how the human brain is wired to cope. Ask any woman who has given birth more than once. However, this lack of memory and denial from my brain did not help my poor physical body that had just about had enough of this and was staging flash daytime sleep attacks: I was perilously close to becoming narcoleptic.

And if that was not enough, you could add schizophrenic to the list. There was the sensible me that went through the surgery and the bad days of chemo, rested when I needed to and listened to good advice. And there was the silly me who did the challenges and the writing. The problem was that the silly me did not know when to stop and the sensible me had to tell it off frequently. So after a delicious lunch, I was packed back off to bed for an afternoon nap. When I awoke, I was offered a nice cup of tea. Oddly, it appeared to taste of elderflower.

This was unsurprising when you understand the increasing number of smaller hoops my family and partner had to jump through daily to appease a health-obsessed me on a mission to rid my body of cancer.

It all started in the morning with a bowl of porridge (organic whole oats, of course, no microwave allowed) and blueberries. This trick was picked up from Bruce Forsyth, who credits his longevity to porridge and precisely 12 blueberries each morning. I also got a nice cup of tea with rice milk as I am dairy free, sort of.

This might seem reasonably easy to you, but when we had a dozen water bottles delivered daily by my mum or dad as they have a fancy water filter which takes out the bad stuff and puts back in the good stuff, this is by no means an easy task. We have red and white wine, sparkling water, elderflower and any bottle my dad has recycled to fill up with healthy water, so it is a bit of a game in our house remembering the true contents of the bottles. However, that morning, the system went wrong when the bottle my partner emptied into the kettle was, in fact, elderflower which – I can tell you from experience – does not taste nice boiled and served up as tea!

Here's a flavour of the challenging diets my devoted family had to wrestle with over the months.

My diet lists

1. Pre-diagnosis – the 'I think I have IBS' diet (basically, nothing with seeds).

2. Post-diagnosis – the 'no red meat, sugar or dairy product' diet (see colon cancer statistics on Western versus African/Eastern diets for proof).

3. Post colon surgery – the low-residue diet to allow the bowel to heal for one month, followed by a high-residue diet a month later (ideally, five small meals a day).

4. Post liver surgery – the 'homemade hearty vegetarian soup as a meal' diet.

5. Recovery and present-day diet – vegetarian with a bit of fish and chicken, plus, for extra fun, cross-referred with the anti-cancer diet and the alkalizing diet with a healthy dose of mucilaginous food (okra, parsley, ginger, linseed and fenugreek seeds).

Now you still might think that sounds pretty fair. But factor in two children, one of whom doesn't think he has eaten unless there is something red and oozing blood on his plate. The other, a vegetarian, insists on baking cakes at the exact time dinner is being prepared. It did not end there. The high-tech cooker hob that my parents had bought me had decided to pack up which meant that someone had to cook all meals needed for three weeks until a replacement was sent on a two-ring gas cooker. (No microwaves please after a Swiss food scientist called Dr Hans-Ulrich Hertel discovered that eating microwave food can potentially cause changes in the blood associated with disease … I could go on.)

And finally, would you please coordinate the arrival of three separate meals with my pill regime: I needed to take chemo tablets with food at eight-hourly intervals. And relax. Oh no, sorry, you can't, you have ironing now to do on account of me still not being able to lift anything heavier than a kettle. High maintenance, me? Say one word and I will throw said kettle at you!

Seriously, there is a lot of sensible advice on anti-cancer diets out there, and I particularly recommend *Anticancer: A New Way of Life* by David Servan-Schreiber.

* * *

Now for the good news and the bad news. I was due to start the second cycle of chemo on the day the NHS nurses and doctors decided to go on strike. This would have meant crossing over a picket line, but after seeing my oncologist in the afternoon, my white blood cell count was too low to continue, so chemo was cancelled. My doctor – we shall call him Dr Needles – was to blood what Paganini was to violins. My blood practically sang as it came out, and I never had any problems satisfying his demand for multiple test tubes of blood.

However, he had no control over the quality of my blood, and I left disappointed to hit delays so early on in my treatment. It did mean that I had an extra week off to try and get the little deserters to come back and fight. But I was feeling really tired and quite reasonably upset about this.

This early capitulation meant that I was now a candidate for injections to stimulate my white blood cells. Unfortunately, they came with a new set of side effects, including bone pain. I was trying not to feel let down, but my body was not coping well with chemo – or, with the immortal words of my laid-back oncologist, the Cheshire Cat: 'If I continue with treatment this week, I may kill you!' Which he said and then went bright red and hooted with laughter, before opening the door and releasing me into a world festering with biological weapons of Rachel destruction.

At the beginning of my chemo regime, some people were concerned about my general laid-backness and had mistaken it for denial, wondering what I was really feeling as I was obviously not doing my fair bit of mourning or raging. As I have already said, anger is not really my thing.

I recognized this worry as the 'there but for the grace of God' syndrome. I had it myself when colleagues or relatives got ill. You cannot imagine how you would deal with something so major and assume the poor soul has courage beyond your wildest dreams or nightmares.

So here is the good news should you ever have any bad news: it is not true! You would almost certainly cope with it the same as me. I have had the honour of meeting some incredible men and women going through similar treatments as well as those in remission. Without exception, they were all getting on with it and living without the heavy burden of 'Why me?' dragging them down. These wonderful people made it easy for me to follow, and I was enormously grateful for them for giving me a crash induction course into the cancer club when I became a recruit. Most of us, however, do get a bit conflicted when we hear 'You fought it' or 'So brave, so inspirational' quotes attached to almost anyone going through cancer. Yes, you probably do get quite brave. Not out of choice but out of necessity. And don't for a minute think that anyone who does not make it through fought any less, or was any less brave or inspirational.

The body and brain are designed to cope better with reality than 'whatifery'. So living and curing yourself becomes a full-time occupation and leaves little space for your brain to indulge in much else.

I have never been one for taking things too seriously, and I found that cancer only encouraged that character trait in me. I am not saying everyone will deal with it in the same way, but the more people realize that the harder burden, by far, is for those watching, caring and worrying for you, the better. I have plenty of people doing this for me, so it would be a complete duplication of tasks to add myself to that list.

Things you can do when you have cancer

1. You have your own 'get out of jail free' card and can behave as badly as you like and get away with anything shy of murder!
   (Although it is very difficult to have the 'satisfaction' of a proper argument with anyone as most people are somewhat loathe, oddly enough, to pick a fight with anyone suffering from cancer.)

2. You can sleep when you want, watch what you want, say what you want.

3. You can send purchases back outside of the 30-day rule and blame chemo. The same goes for parking tickets.

4. You can ignore all emails.

➔

5. You don't need to shave your legs or pluck your eyebrows.

6. You get your own way in arguments (see 1.).

7. You can get out of having to buy heaps of Christmas presents.

Things you cannot do when you have cancer

1. You cannot get affordable travel insurance easily. (I was quoted over £4,000 for a week in Ibiza.)

2. You cannot continue to highlight your hair when you are on certain chemo drugs: there will not be any hair to highlight.

3. You are unable to listen to others moaning about their job/life/hair/salary/holidays, and so on.

4. You cannot take out a mortgage or life insurance.

5. You cannot join Match.com with confidence!

* * *

Throughout my treatment, I have noticed that doctors often say one thing and mean something else entirely. In my experience, the medical profession falls into two camps: those who have the greatest respect for potential risk and would not be out of place in the accountancy or legal profession and those who think that Bear Grylls could do with toughening up a bit. The trick is to be able to cotton on quickly which one you are dealing with and ratchet up or down their advice accordingly.

I am keeping a running list for my own amusement, but let me share some of it with you ...

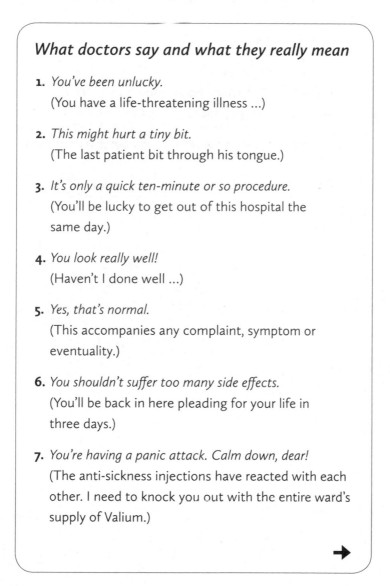

What doctors say and what they really mean

1. *You've been unlucky.*
   (You have a life-threatening illness ...)

2. *This might hurt a tiny bit.*
   (The last patient bit through his tongue.)

3. *It's only a quick ten-minute or so procedure.*
   (You'll be lucky to get out of this hospital the same day.)

4. *You look really well!*
   (Haven't I done well ...)

5. *Yes, that's normal.*
   (This accompanies any complaint, symptom or eventuality.)

6. *You shouldn't suffer too many side effects.*
   (You'll be back in here pleading for your life in three days.)

7. *You're having a panic attack. Calm down, dear!*
   (The anti-sickness injections have reacted with each other. I need to knock you out with the entire ward's supply of Valium.)

➡

8. *You're a bit poorly.*
   (Cancel all engagements for the rest of the year.)

9. *It's possible, just about possible that we can reverse this one day.*
   (Don't sue me if we can't.)

10. *You have a needle phobia.*
    (All your veins have collapsed, and I really don't want to put in yet another canula.)

11. *The pharmacy will be up with your drugs in a couple of hours.*
    (Don't book the taxi home until tomorrow!)

Perseverance is not a long race;
it is many short races one after the other.

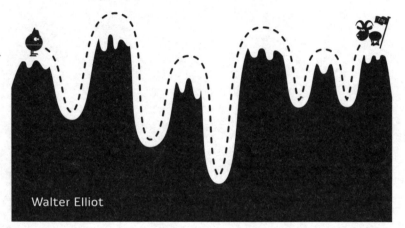

Walter Elliot

CHAPTER TWELVE

*

More chemo adventures

Most families are content to be found in shops or, worse still, estate agents in an attempt to empty the contents of their bank accounts before bunkering down for the relaxing budget festival we call Christmas.

However, my family and friends decided this year that there was absolutely no way they were going to eat Christmas dinner without first emptying the contents and cavities of their bodies and descended like a flash mob on hospitals around the country as a precaution.

While their hospital results were all in the 'good news' category and bladders and colons were all flushed out and ready for action, my white blood cells had just about managed to scrape through to the minimum level for chemo to go ahead on the appointed day.

As I may have hinted earlier, my family has low-boredom thresholds unsullied from a lifetime of watching TV. So any chance to join me in hospital was billed as the outing of the week and well worth bartering for. My mother won that week, after promising to do everyone's Christmas shopping as payment for her reward.

You may also remember that I was the last one to leave the ward and turn off the lights on chemo round number one, so I naturally assumed that I had done my time and would be fast-tracked through the system on the day.

Not so. Dr Deputy Needles (aka the Hairdresser), in his gratitude to find some blood from one of my damaged veins the previous day (we had got used to checking on my blood a day beforehand to avoid turning up and being constantly turned away from the chemo ward at the last minute) and temporary blinded by his success, completely overlooked the demands from the chemo vampires for two test tubes prior to starting chemo. He was nicknamed the Hairdresser on account of his conversational tactics which relied solely on asking me where I was going for my holiday this year. I could not decide whether he was being ironic or serious.

Anyway, the chemo ward overlooked this as well until about half an hour after kick-off when all hell broke loose. Thankfully, Carol, one of the sweet chemo nurses, who managed to combine gentle compassion with an organizational zeal unmatched even by the North Koreans, was on the case.

More blood was demanded, and after an hour or two's wait for the test to check that my kidneys and liver were still doing whatever it is liver and kidneys do, she plugged me into my USB port for that day's 'special', Oxaliplatin. The happy hour lasted two hours.

While I was waiting for the side effects to hit, I was distracted by one of the other customers at our alternative cocktail bar who reminded me that however rubbish we feel, we don't have far to look to find someone worse off. Alerted by her unique walking style, I discovered that this brave and cheerful lady had had no less than five knee replacements and three shoulder replacements. Now, even in my drugged state, I was able to ascertain that this poor woman had gone through knees and shoulders faster than I go through a pair of leggings. And now she was back in suffering from lymphoma, starting her first chemo regime and about to break the news that night to her 92-year-old father. A sobering thought.

As I watched the chairs emptying and the nurses leaving, my mum offered to give the ward a once-over with the duster and Hoover, before turning off the lights and going home to await the fun chemo number two had in store for me.

Not content to let me rest on my laurels, the second chemo round added a new menu of side effects, including a frozen face, nose, forehead and eyes – like plastic surgery without the benefits. To boot, it caused some funny gazes at parents' evening.

My legs had also chosen to play up this time, with constant pains in my shins and pins and needles all the way up whenever my body temperature dropped below room temperature. I may have brought some of the new side effects on myself by reducing my steroids which made me jumpy, insomniac and tearful. The pay-off was a miserable three days of feeling really sick when I could barely keep down water. I made a mental note not to play around with steroids in future.

Make sure you ask your oncologist for one of the following anti-sickness drugs (the best ones are not always offered up front). Chemotherapy is famous for inducing nausea and vomiting, also referred to as CINV (chemo-induced nausea and vomiting). This is because chemo can injure the stomach cells that start off the process of being or feeling sick. It can directly activate the area of the brain responsible for producing nausea and vomiting. There is a long list of anti-sickness drugs that you need to experiment with as they work on different receptors in the brain.

1. **Benzamides** such as Metoclopramide blocks the effects of dopamine on the areas of the brain signalling vomiting. It also speeds up the emptying of your stomach, so you can get diarrhoea afterwards.

2. **Serotonin antagonists** are most commonly prescribed and include Ondansetron which blocks the effects of Serotonin on the vomiting centres in both the brain and the intestines.

3. **Corticosteroids**, also called steroids, such as Dexamethasone, can interfere with sleeping, but help with nausea.

4. **Benzodiazepines** include Lorazepam and Nozanin (Levomepromazine). These tranquillizers are used to treat anxiety disorders, but can be powerful because they calm down the brain. They also help with sleeping.

The two antiemetics that worked best for me (and I imagine cost enough to bankrupt the Primary Care Trust as they appear to be offered as a last resort) were Emend and Nozanin. Emend apparently works well to treat 'anticipatory' nausea and vomiting and blocks a substance in the body called Neurokinin.

One drug I never got to try was Nabilone, which is made from cannabis. It is used for treating severe sickness from chemo that other drugs cannot reach.

* * *

When bits of the Sly Old Fox started growing out of control and needed removing, I had no idea this illness would lead me to a bunch of people whose daily motivation is truly beyond me – people who find reserves of kindness and generosity of time when everyone else is flying around at increasing speeds in preparation for the annual 24-hour shut-down we call Christmas.

Hopeful Notes is a non-profit local music society led by Tom Van Kaenel whose aim is to help and heal through music. The people involved gave up every lunch hour before Christmas to perform carols in the Churchill Hospital in aid of bowel cancer. This was even more remarkable as I only had the pleasure of meeting Tom recently, and I am sure these volunteers all had charities that were closer to their hearts. But their heartfelt singing not only gave a necessary lift to the patients, visitors and staff, but encouraged people to donate generously to charity. I do find this amazing, and I can only conclude that, from my experience, the more austere our circumstances and depressing the news is, the more this is countered and exceeded by the growing pool of kindness, positivity and generosity. Tom has since spent 77 days cycling from the West Coast to the East Coast of the USA raising money for service members, veterans and their families from the UK and the US through his charity Sea2Sea. What a guy. I was also encouraged, despite my low mood at the time, by the ever-growing army of volunteers I had access to. I had a new therapist courtesy of the Sunrise Cancer Unit in High Wycombe. Apparently, I was eligible for four free treatments, and I chose reflexology from one of the generous volunteers. It was the most blissful way to spend an hour after my chemo regime, and I really think it helped with some of my side effects. I did not even mind Carol coming in afterwards to land a needle in my stomach to encourage the bone marrow to fire up!

This was followed by my wonderful regular Reiki therapist Mary Holloway, another volunteer, who has been treating me since the beginning. She was always full of useful information and tips to help me accept my situation and feel less nervous about all the random things going on in my body. This angel was sent to me by the Rennie Grove cancer charity as part of their Hospice at Home care, and very welcome it was, too.

However, my Reiki session that afternoon was not quite what Mary was aiming for as she pressed play on her relaxation tape and asked me to breathe in peace and love and breathe out fear and tension.

The assault on my senses did not match previous sessions where a kaleidoscope of colours danced in front of my eyes.

The first clue that relaxation might be an elusive goal was the arrival of three boys on bikes who galloped two stairs at a time into my son's bedroom. I have heard rutting stags make less noise. I breathed in deeper, my diaphragm emptying fast. 'Keep the noise down, please,' I begged. A moment's silence followed by the bedroom door shutting and then sounds of the punch bag being knocked into next door's hallway and more sounds of cats being neutered. Why are boys not taught in science that three inches of MDF does not cover them in a cloak of silence?

The doorbell rang, announcing the arrival of my mother: 'JOSEPH, THERE ARE SIX PAIRS OF SHOES BLOCKING THE DOOR, I CAN'T GET IN!' Two more children, one of them mine, fell in behind her. The dog barked. The phone rang. The boys fell over each other to get down the stairs first. Joseph began his earnest attempt to play *Mad World* loudly and repetitively, and the poor strains of Mary's relaxation tape finally gave up their feeble attempt to distract and started to wail disconcertingly. We both collapsed into giggles and gave up.

In the space of 30 minutes we had moved from a relaxed family house to a lunatic asylum without the usual familiar interval of a mad hatter's tea party. Mary told me the Reiki would still do its work even if I was unable to benefit from the normal levels of relaxation and made a mental note never to turn up again outside of school hours.

* * *

Another unexpected pleasure during my chemo break was a friendship with a wonderfully warm and charming scientist, Dr Robin Hesketh, a cancer biologist of some repute who has worked at the Department of Biochemistry at the University of Cambridge for over 25 years. He was in the process of publishing his latest book called *Betrayed by Nature: The War on Cancer*. Recognizing the need for a blog to promote his book, he approached me.

In Robin's words: 'She was looking for distraction from embarking on post-surgical chemotherapy for bowel cancer. As a virgin blogger, I was desperate for someone experienced to tell me what to do. In traditional male fashion, my overtures were very much of the hope rather than anticipation variety – even with my manic enthusiasm for cells and molecules I had to admit that someone grappling with colorectal carcinoma might find less than irresistible the post of Reviewing Editor (unpaid) for articles on cancer. But no, she said yes! She stuck by her word by marking my first essay – with disconcerting perception – within 24 hours (university tutors please note!). And in the process we have become the best of friends.'

Now science (or, in this case, Dr Hesketh) needs me as

much as my dog needs a manicure. I can certainly testify that the distraction was well worth the odd suggestion I made to put a picture in here or there. But we struggled through, and I learnt more in those months than I learnt in all the years I was interned at school. Robin had produced, in his words, a SciNov, a book that reads like a novel in which science and the folk that do it make the story. It is a wonderful book, and I heartily recommend it, as well as his blog, of course. Check it out on: www.cancerforall.wordpress.com

Here are just a few titbits I learnt from reading Robin's book about cancer.

1. Cancer is nothing more than an abnormal growth of cells caused by mutation – a sort of genetic roulette.

2. Stress can affect cancer – apparently, the two most stressful things for us are a) making a speech and b) doing arithmetic in front of an audience (five minutes of these is enough to push our salivary cortisol levels up two- to four-fold).

3. Cortisol suppresses the immune system and reduces the number of white cells in the blood.

4. Cancers come about because changes in the DNA code (mutations) affect how proteins work, or even whether they are made at all. You cannot catch a cancer gene. Something goes wrong along the way and turns our cells into delinquents. That is not to say that some unlucky souls are born with a bad genetic deal in the form of a mutation that makes them cancer prone.

5. It is a biological balancing act between controlling the accelerators (the abnormally active genes called oncogenes) and the brakes (the tumour suppressor genes).

6. It is incredible that cancer happens at all when you understand the genetic mayhem. (Robin describes it a bit like a building-block model of the Eiffel Tower being the target of a child's tantrum, reducing it to a jumble of unconnected blocks. And from this mess, a cell has to cobble together enough of the 'blueprint for life' to enable it to carry on and still be able to function.)

7. If we all lived to be 140, we would all get cancer. In fact, getting cancer young is most unlucky, and we are classed as 'outriders' statistically. About 2,000 people under 50 get bowel cancer each year which might be a small number compared to the 41,000 people in the UK *per annum*, but it is significant and growing.

* * *

Those of you who know me will nod enthusiastically when I say I have a lifelong obsession with arriving anywhere late. But even I was disappointed with myself when I was sent home again from the chemo ward and told to return the following week when my white blood cells were up to the job in hand.

Yes, I am afraid I was neutropenic again. Neutropenia, a decrease in the number of neutrophils (the most important white blood cells), was becoming such a regular event in my life that I did not even need to check the spelling. But if you are interested, it meant that my neutrophils, or neuts as the medical profession fondly call them, which are the defenders in my white blood cells that foreign bodies usually run into first, were down again.

It would be charitable to say it did not hurt too much when Dr Deputy Needles unsuccessfully tried three times to get blood out of my damaged veins that morning when doing the normal checks of my blood levels prior to starting chemo. After an hour or so plugged into the saline drip, the results came back with red ink all over them and a note to try harder.

There was evidence mounting to suggest that my neutrophils were pacifists and were no more interested in fighting these cancer cells than I was in going to the Boxing Day sales (I would rather sit on the sofa with a nice cup of tea). So, in addition to the bone marrow injections I enjoyed to encourage activity, I could now add selenium and Resbid tablets to my regime, two cups of green tea a day, a partridge in a pear tree and a diet so high in protein that I expected to get offered automatic membership to the World Boxing Federation.

Looking for positives, I had a week off over Christmas to spend with the kids before they went back to school feeling *relatively* normal. Then I thought that it was time for a serious word with the Cheshire Cat, my oncologist, to decide on the path of lesser risk: delaying each cycle for another week or reducing this early on to chemo for cowards? I thought even he would relent from his usual 'let's see how it goes' response and dream up some new delicious-sounding chemicals to test-drive.

* * *

I could not help feeling nervous: 2011 had been such a year of change and upheaval that, as New Year's Eve approached, I felt sure there was still time to pack in at least one more major event.

I suppose I was not the only one who saw 2011 as a year of fear, and I was lucky enough to miss a great chunk of it by turning off the news for at least three months while dealing with my own 'event of the year'. So much had happened that it was impossible to remember it all. And as I successfully managed to avoid some of the worse incidents, I cleverly decided not to read the annual roundup across the media as I did not want to accidently stumble across something I had missed and had to squeeze in all that worry into a few hours or risk it leaking into a brand new 2012.

On my own micro level, I would like to rewrite 2011 as a year when I learnt the power of love, extreme kindness and generosity, and so I decided to greet the new year with a cheery smile and a plan to be 100 per cent healthier, 50 per cent tidier, 25 per cent slower and 25 per cent more tolerant, because 2012 was not going anywhere until at least 2013 – and that felt a very long time away.

I was pondering if it says something about the English that, despite the richness of our vocabulary which allows us to draw shades of distinction unavailable to non-English speakers, I could find only a couple of words to express thank you. (For the record, Eskimos have 50 words for types of snow and Italians have over 500 names for different types of pasta.) Right at that moment it did not seem in any way enough for me to express my gratitude to everyone who had got me this far and was still looking like they had legs to get me through the rest of the pitiful 'journey'.

* * *

I started the New Year back on track. Neutropenia was on hold for the time being.

The only benefit of being neutropenic had been the extra week off to try and build the white blood cells back up. The Cheshire Cat informed me in a matter-of-fact way that week that I had lazy bone marrow – something I could not help feeling rather guilty about.

But what a treat those extra two weeks had been! I spent literally days forgetting about having cancer and feeling ill and enjoyed the sensations in my body as they were reawakened. Believe me, it is pretty wonderful to be able to think in a joined-up way, talk, smell anything (although not the dog), taste and sleep. There is nothing more euphoric than feeling well again once the chemo fog has lifted and you can see and feel clearly. I felt like a blind man learning to see.

Unfortunately, this respite into normalness was short-lived, and I was soon in again starting chemo cycle number three.

If you are inviting a toxic cocktail of chemicals into your body, that have the power of life and death, it is quite within the realms of plausibility to expect a trade-off in the form of feeling crap. And so I spent the following week or so running at around 25 per cent of my normal 'me-ness'.

I arrived at the Sunrise Centre determined to practise mindfulness after having seen a BBC report promoting the success of happiness and removal of pain. But this also was short-lived as I was approached to enter a national research study into colorectal cancer and was asked nicely if I would care to give them some blood for this study. As I already had the portacath tube plugged into my jugular, it seemed rude not to, and I let the nurse take a couple of test tubes. They are still recruiting for this study and, at the time, had about 20,000 people, but needed 30,000. It may be a little while before we see the results of the link between genetics and bowel cancer, something that is very close to our family's heart (or should I say bowels?).

Momentarily distracted from my meditation, I looked around for suitable reading material and finding only 'Caught out! I facebooked my boyfriend and found his wife!', I decided to read the nice brochures on side effects for my latest panacea – a perky little drug that promised to eradicate both insomnia and sickness. However, on reading the promotional material I was alarmed to find that these Nozanin tablets were commonly used to treat schizophrenia. Was there something my doctor wasn't telling me?

* * *

This 'dalliance' with normal life over Christmas allowed me and my brother David to put together a tender for challenge number two. (Challenge number one had been to play the piano in a Christmas concert at the Churchill dressed as a Banana Giraffe.) A real humdinger of a challenge.

And we got a feeling that it was not going to be as simple as it first seemed! David had written the following on my blog when I was too ill to post anything.

A search for 'architects with experience building 40ft giraffes on residential properties' returned zero results in Google. (And they say you can find just about anything online?)

We're assuming a giraffe, real or otherwise, is a highly technical piece of building that we can't just trust to any fly-by-night architect … so we're going for the best-of-the-best of famous award-winning UK architects. It'll be a 10-way pitch situation, so we've put together a request for designs.

May the best architect (with no previous experience of building 40ft giraffes on residential properties) win.

This is a copy of the brief which we sent out and the reply. (No alcohol was consumed during this process.)

9 January, 2012

Dear Architect,

We would formally like you to present ideas for the project attached.

Your earliest response is appreciated.

With best regards,

Rachel Bown

Banana Giraffes

Section 1: About Banana Giraffes
Section 2: What this is
Section 3: The opportunity
Section 4: The brief
Section 5: Your fee and deadlines
Section 6: Legal

Section 1: About Banana Giraffes

Hello.

My name is Rachel Bown, thanks for reading this far.
I'm 45, and was diagnosed with bowel cancer last year.
I am currently in the midst of chemotherapy.

To keep myself from going completely stir-crazy, I have set myself a few challenges to raise awareness and as much

➡

money as I can for a bowel cancer charity. (The statistics in Section 3 are real figures of a cancer that could do with more awareness and early diagnosis and treatment.)

My first challenge was more on a personal level: performing a piano recital at the Churchill Hospital in Oxford. It went well, we raised a bit of money and it was covered by the BBC locally.

This challenge is a different one, but one that has the chance for greater publicity, and the BBC has already agreed to cover any significant milestones on the way to getting permission to erect a 40ft banana giraffe from my house.

Do I really expect to get a 40ft banana giraffe sticking out of my house? When we first came up with the idea, I thought it would be some kind of joke, but now I am getting strangely set on seeing it through. Whatever happens, with the help of all the people involved and with publicity through the charity, it is sure to generate a lot of interest and, hopefully, donations.

I would hugely appreciate a response of any kind. I would even more hugely appreciate a response that included drawings and concepts. It would be phenomenal if you got involved with this idea and helped see it through in whatever way you can.

With many thanks,
Rachel Bown

PS: I currently have a blog over at www.bananagiraffes. com where you can find some more information ... and stuff.

→

Section 2: What this is

A fee-paying pitch (see envelope enclosed) for the best UK-based designs possible for the brief in Section 4.

What we would like to see:

i) Initial designs, for the brief in Section 4, in your preferred format (model, sketch, digital visualization). These are in no way binding (see Section 6), but should be highly conceptual interpretations of the brief.

ii) Rough timelines and project management proposals.

iii) Any proposals for working with partners and your relationship with them.

iv) Costs for the consultation phase, the design phase and overseeing the build phase. Plus any necessary maintenance work required on an annual basis.

v) Short biographies of key people involved.

vi) Short case studies of similar work undertaken. In particular, those entailing successful negotiations on convention-challenging work with planning bodies.

Each section above is allocated unique points and weighting. These can be made available to you on request.

Section 3: The opportunity

We believe the brief (Section 4) has the potential to increase not only annual revenue but also positive international brand awareness for the successful architects.

At Banana Giraffes, we inhabit a positive mind-space

➡

and have increasingly large brand presence in a growing market (40,000 in the UK alone, growing at a UK rate of 110 people every day. Global audience increased by 1.24 million in 2008).

Our brand attributes are: vision, positivity, optimism and fun.

You have been chosen as you match one if not all of them.

Section 4: The brief

The project is to construct a 40ft banana giraffe at a residential property in Holmer Green, Buckinghamshire.

No information can be given as to what a banana giraffe is. This is a conceptual challenge and should be met creatively.

Local planning regulations have been checked and no section can be found containing guidance for constructing 40ft banana giraffes. We take this as positive news although it may be wise to expect heavy resistance.

Should you accept this challenge, please do contact me at Rachel@bananagiraffes.com

Section 5: Your fee and timelines

There are no restrictions on budget.

The amount chargeable by yourselves should be set by yourselves.

All money made by yourselves should be donated directly to the registered charity, Beating Bowel Cancer, minus any costs for sandwiches (restricted to £50 total).

➡

The £50 sandwich fee should be paid directly to my mother for any sandwiches she makes for yourselves in the course of the project.

She makes great sandwiches from quality ingredients.

Sandwiches made by my mother will be charged at cost to yourselves.

This section on sandwiches is not intended to be a distraction from any other information in this section and you should pay little attention to it.

Timelines are good. We like them very much, and they should be coloured in the colour of the Banana Giraffes' brand – yellow.

Section 6: Legal

Being of an optimistic and trusting nature, we cannot foresee any legal problems at all and have left this bit blank.

The only problems we could possibly see would be about the sandwiches bit in Section 5, but you can leave this bit out.

Banana Giraffes pitch Jan, 2012

I admit that not all architectural practices are designed with a funny bone in mind. But we hit gold with David Chipperfield Architects, who possessed not only a fully flexible funny bone but also a heart of gold. Their kind letter of reply is shown opposite. Sadly, we are still waiting for the giraffe to be built.

David Chipperfield Architects

11 York Road, London SE1 7NX

17 February, 2012

Dear Rachel,

Thank you for your letter of 9 January regarding your request to achieve a 40ft banana giraffe projecting from the top of your house.

Congratulations on your imagination, energy and ambition – not to mention your ability to completely confound us. We really don't know where to begin with such a task.

Whilst we try to get our collective minds around your mission, please find enclosed a donation to Beating Bowel Cancer.

Thanks again for thinking of us. Your energy and approach is an inspiration.

Regards

Andrew Phillips
for David Chipperfield Architects

*   *   *

I had the rarest of days and went for a girly lunch on my birthday at my parents' house. It was a real super-sized tonic. As I was not sure until the day whether I would be well enough, my best friend Jenny organized the lunch with five seconds' notice. After a few 'you look better than I thought' rituals and the passing of cards bearing giraffe motives, I did a quick radio interview with my new best radio friend Malcolm Boyden from BBC Oxford. Malcolm wanted an update on the growth of a giraffe out of the roof of my house. Then it was down to a lunch fit for a forever-changing-her-mind cancer diva!

Jenny, I have decided, is the type of person who is impossible not to obey, and I am sure everyone who meets her must fall under her spell and agree to anything she says. On my birthday, she pulled together the most delicious of meals with more ease than I could display unwrapping a supermarket sandwich.

The day went so well that I did not even notice myself slipping down the hill of the forties mountain and into the next survey bracket.

The week continued to be a good week. A very good week. A terribly kind friend of David had given me five tickets for his box at the Royal Albert Hall to see Cirque du Soleil during half term. He said it would do me good as it was an inspirational show of strength and courage. I have said it before, and I will say it again, I am a very spoilt girl!

Keeping up with my promise to try new experiences, I followed that by enjoying the pleasure of lying down for half an hour each week covered in ultrafine needles, courtesy of another medic to add to my list – an acupuncturist.

This was not as painful as it sounded, but I am naturally disappointed that I left the session without having given at least a test tube of blood. It turned out he was not your average

Dracula. Keen observers of *Qi* may not be surprised to hear that mine was blocked and in need of a good old flushout and rebalancing. While this was all supposed to help with the nausea and the white blood cell problem, an excellent by-product of all this was a clear head. I had energy! It might still have been like a typical journey to Kingston, fast, slow, fast, slow, stop, crash, but I sincerely hoped to see more success with removing my roadblocks than I would expect from the three motorways I used to have the pleasure of travelling on every day.

Observing that the biggest obstacle to getting properly well might be the nonsense that still circulated in my head, the acupuncturist gave me a good talking to about tapping into the power of my mind. I left with the following two challenges that I was to do at every opportunity.

1. I had to imagine lying on a golden blanket and, starting from the top of my head, breathe in white light from the universe, feeling it purifying and cleansing every cell in my body from the top of my head to the tip of my toes, concentrating for longer on my liver and intestines. A kind of holistic CT scan, I guess.

2. I had to practise drinking a cup of green tea slowly, tasting every mouthful, smelling the tea, feeling the warmth on my face and concentrating on nothing else than the sensation of drinking and the feel of the new bone china cup. I also needed to apply this to the task of eating a meal.

This was a far cry from my usual practice of eating and drinking while on the computer, watching TV and talking on the phone, all at the same time and at speeds that would make a hamster feel giddy.

If I could do all this and keep my sense of humour, he prescribed a regular jolly good laugh, although, of course, not while eating or meditating.

* * *

I cannot leave it there without thanking the people who gave birth to me all those winters ago (I am now 46 winters old) and who are putting up with the consequences now.

My mum – how awe-inspiring can one woman be? She has been my rock, my best friend, my comfort all my life. I wish everyone had a mother like mine (but not mine, so hands off!). I have been asked countless times to 'lend' her out over the years, and she sometimes does go on missions, but always comes back. She is with me on my dark days, when none of you really know, and she celebrates my up days, too. She is best friend to my friends, mother to my kids; she cleans and hoovers, brings water and food, takes the children home at the drop of a hat and stays strong when she herself has been through hell and back. I will never find anyone in my life like my mother!

And my dad – what compassion and generosity! My wonderful dad has done more to eradicate my cancer than any person I know would – from research to taking his very own air miles and travelling to Hungary to pick up a suitcase full of cancer drugs from a woman he knew remotely. He reads and studies all the time for new things to help me; he books and pays for nutritionists and acupuncturists, pills and potions and anything else he can get his hands on. He brings me daily nutritious juices which he juices himself and drives like fury to get them to me within the 20-minute optimum drinking time. I have not yet found an hour early enough to get up to catch my dad out! Waitresses, therapists and shops around the country will testify to the physical battles that take place over payment everywhere we go. I have not won yet, and I am 29 years younger than him and in full-time employment …

Every time anyone says, 'You're very brave, how do you do it?', I refer them to the above. I love them to bits and am very blessed.

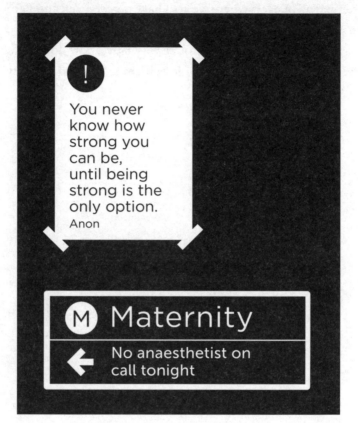

CHAPTER THIRTEEN

✳

Approaching the end of chemo

In view of the 'Be loud, be clear' awareness week that culminated with the launch of the government's first TV campaign for bowel cancer, I would like to emphasize that early detection is a matter of life or death. We need to get to grips with this embarrassment about all things bowel and help knock bowel cancer off its unwelcome Top 2 slot for cancer deaths in the UK. We lag behind the rest of the world, so something is going wrong in this genteel island, methinks …

It is high time we were louder and clearer about what is going on with our bums and go and see our doctor urgently if we are suffering from the following symptoms for three weeks or more:

1. *Bleeding from the bottom without any obvious reason*
You may also notice other symptoms such as straining, soreness, lumps and itchiness around the back passage. Often, this is caused by piles, but it is also a 'red flag' symptom for urgent

investigation, so do go and see your GP who can take a full history and do an initial examination.

2. *A persistent change in bowel habits*
Any unexpected or unexplained change to your normal habits of going to the toilet and emptying your bowels is a cause for concern. Sometimes, you may have problems with constipation and have the physical feeling that your bowel is not completely empty. It is especially important to go and make a doctor's appointment if you are going to the toilet more often than usual or are experiencing looser stools and/or passing lots of clear, jelly-like mucus.

3. *Abdominal pain*
This may be constant or will come and go. Seek help immediately if it becomes severe.

4. *A lump in your tummy*
You should pay particular attention if the lump is on the right-hand side.

5. *Unexplained tiredness, dizziness and breathlessnes*
These may indicate anaemia as your colon is unable to use the food you eat to its full potential.

6. *Unexpected and unexplained weight loss*
Have it checked out by your doctor straight away.

* * *

It is incredible how many people congratulate you and say, well done, you are halfway through. Yet at the time, I could not join in with the premature celebrations. But off I went again for chemo cycle number four after two blood tests to make sure my white blood cells were conquering their fear, standing up straight and defending their stations with more than the usual feeble 'say no to cancer' placards. So imagine my shock when they passed their physical for the first time ever that morning. What heroes! I can only assume they were watching *Birdsong* on Sunday with me, or maybe it was the bone marrow injections, the acupuncture or the new pills which I had been gagging on all month.

The day before the Cheshire Cat, confronted with my lazy bone marrow and a growing list of side effects, had decided it was time to lower the dose by 20 per cent.

Jenny was my chemo caddy and kept the whole ward amused by 'Jenny TV' as I called her when she was in entertainment mode. She also did a good job of alarming my chemo nurse by explaining how we met: 'We worked together, fell in love and then … when did we have our children, Rachel?' My nurse nearly dropped my medication in shock and now had us down as a couple.

* * *

After a couple of weeks, I was leaving my latest persistent vegetative state, and my activity tolerance rose to an impressive 30 minutes, which meant that I could turn back my attention to observing the strange and funny ways in which my life and, in particular, my appearance had changed.

Speaking as someone who would rather step willingly onto a flying saucer than a set of scales, I was finding this new monitoring and obsession with my weight alarming.

The only other time I recall my weight being under such scrutiny was during and after pregnancy, and I have done my best since to forget and unlearn kilograms should I ever accidently fall onto any scales again. However, I was now weighed more frequently than an average bag of goodies on *MasterChef*, and it appeared that I had eaten the contents, too.

But what I could not quite comprehend was the look of glee in the nurse's eye when the scales topped the last chemo session, and she exclaimed, 'Well done, you've put on weight, go on treat yourself to a fried Eccles cake sandwich.' Such is the way of the chemo nurses who have mastered the art of making the depressing reality of the chemo ward seem mundane and pretty normal that they think this calls for some serious celebration.

Another interesting thing I noticed was that I did not conform to what people thought a cancer patient should look like. I know looking 'hot' had different connotations, and it seemed awfully vain to worry about my appearance while I was daily ingesting enough chemicals to deep-clean the bathing facilities at a senior boys school. I did feel guilty for looking so 'ruddy' when I saw people's reaction and, for a fleeting moment, worried that they thought I was putting it all on. And yet again, I felt a twinge of guilt for assuming in the past that your outer appearance is a good indicator of how you are feeling inside.

* * *

I thought we were due an update on the medical research progress of Superdad. Those of you who know my dad will testify to his methodical research and caution and certainly would not label him a shopaholic. But there is a gene in our family that can kick in with no prior warning and cause all manner of contradictions. One notable example of this break from normal service was the purchase of a wild, untamed

New Forest pony bought with about ten minutes' notice for his 10-year-old daughter (me) after driving past a 'For sale' sign during a week's summer holiday. The decision was even more alarming when you consider I knew then as much about horsemanship as Fred Goodwin did about restraint.

Not quite on the same level of spontaneity and enjoyment, but nonetheless caused by the same charming quirk, the shopaholic gene kicked in once again, and we now had more remedies than your flagship Holland & Barrett. The latest purchase to join this collection was Chinese herbs.

To help persuade me to drink this brown potion to treat my blood, Superdad gulped down a glass and declared it tasted very nice and rather like warm liquorice. Meanwhile, Super-mum carried on fumigating the house and had to drink her potion in secret in the kitchen for fear of giving away telltale facial signs of distress. I then drunk mine and while I might need to have my brain thoroughly washed before I view it as a treat, it was not half as bad as I thought.

* * *

It must have been mere days since my last treats, so my dad decided I could do with another top-up and booked me and Jenny into Hartwell House in Buckinghamshire for a couple of days R&R.

As we arrived at Hartwell House for our overnight spa stay, we walked smack bang into a film set. The security guy at the door and the manager ushered us towards the BBC area as we walked into the Grand Hall. It was only quick thinking by Jenny, who alerted the confused duo that we were paying guests, which avoided us causing all manner of mayhem with Jacqueline Bisset and Anthony Head.

The BBC was filming a mini series called *Dancing on the Edge* set in the 1930s and due out in 2013. There were over 80 crew members, lorries galore outside, and filming went on for 12 hours each day, all for four minutes of footage. It was nice to see the BBC doing its bit for the deficit!

Hartwell House, a pretty spectacular place, is perfect for relaxation, especially as all guests obviously take a vow of silence when they check in. You could hear a pin drop, which was a bit of a temptation for Jenny and I to liven up the guests, but after several attempts of CPR they were not to be revived. So we turned our attention on the staff instead, and when asked on an hourly basis if there was anything they could do for us, we came up with a long and inventive list which involved miniature goats in the room, dancing men and horses, a blanket for Molly, the car, and an underground tunnel to the spa building.

These requests were met with good humour and a nod of agreement, and although we had a green flashing alien on the ceiling in our room all night, we never found the miniature goats or champagne-filled bath. We crunched our way through the ice to the spa (Hartwell House recorded temperatures of minus 11 on the day we arrived) and cooked ourselves like seafood in the jacuzzi, lost a couple of stones in the steam room and tried to get a beauty treatment. Unfortunately, they refused to touch anything of me other than my hands on account of the chemotherapy, which they obviously thought was treat enough. So I paid for a manicure and promptly smudged it all off trying to get dressed.

* * *

Chemo is like carrying around a heavy paddling pool full of water. Sensible advice would be to never attempt it on your own. But here I was attempting to do the very same.

Mr partner and I split up. My partner's coping mechanism was to try and take even more control. I began to feel trapped and treated as an invalid as he took over every aspect of my life. I know this was borne out of love and fear. However, it isolated me more and more from the rest of my family and friends who were not only kept away from my bedside, but visits were limited at the house. I was too weak at that stage to complain, but the atmosphere that descended was like a cloud that was so thick and heavy with water that the moss was visible inside and the only thing moving in it were snails. Even my children were nervous and kept their distance.

This continued for several months, with relationships between all of us worsening. This was not me. And it was certainly not the way I wanted to live my life. I had always got energy from other people, and any tiredness I might have felt physically was more than made up for by the mental boost their company gave me.

Early in February, a crisis that had been brewing for a long time erupted and resulted in our relationship finishing abruptly and that very same day. The shock and tears were sickening on both fronts, and I wondered how I would cope alone. Then a wonderful thing happened. People started returning in droves. My house was full of fun and laughter again. The cloud had lifted, and my family and friends moved in to fill the space. I felt lighter mentally and stronger physically.

I was now in the thick of the chemo phase, the hard middle term. And it got me reflecting on the things chemo took from me, but also rather cheekily things I could thank chemo for.

List of things I missed during chemo

1. Thinking about men ... in that way!
   (Particularly ironic to be told by my oncologist that
   using contraception is vitally important during chemo.
   I wanted to talk about life and death, not my sex life ...)

2. Concentration

3. The taste of things, especially white wine and water

4. The thrill of trying on new clothes in changing rooms

5. Seeing the reflection of my old pre-surgery body in
   the mirror

6. My mum and dad staying over at my house, allowing
   me to be a child again
   (For all our sakes, they had to go back to their house
   after the first week, and I had to learn to be on my
   own again.)

7. My blonde hair, the bits where the grey curly roots
   are now

List of things I did not miss during chemo

1. Planning ahead

2. Washing my hair every other day

3. Meetings

4. Action and status notes from meetings

* * *

When we split up, I was thrown back into learning to do lots of things for myself again. To my surprise, I found I liked it! For many years, I had been firmly convinced that there are things which I am hopelessly incapable of doing, and I happily kept topping up this list over the last six months. But there comes a time in your treatment after a long period of enforced abstinence when you actually get excited again by the simple things in life.

For example, I was sure that the novelty of cooking would soon wear off, and my dear mum who was watching in the wings was ready to magic up a meal the minute my energy flagged. But for that moment I was enjoying browsing around a supermarket and thinking of inventive things to do with chickpeas and lentils. I also enjoyed making a fire (after the hot flush of chemo had passed, I usually felt cold), tidying the house and chucking out stuff.

And finally, dipping my toe back into the workplace. This new style of 'working' was most agreeable. It involved popping in to catch up with my team, colleagues and boss. If you have been AWOL for six months, you will get many reactions. The most common are big bear hugs and exclamations of 'You look good!' coupled with the confession 'You looked pretty dog rough before you went off sick but we didn't want to say'.

There are inevitably also a few people who will not meet your eyes and are excruciatingly embarrassed that you are ill and terrified you will want to talk to them about it. And, for goodness sake, it involves bowels! A double no-no.

But the oddest thing is time, a concept I am frequently reminded is hopelessly unreliable for measuring anything, a guaranteed candidate for room 101 if you ask me. For example, the last six months had involved such a dizzyingly fast amount of change and head rewiring that I felt at the very least it was comparable with running a small Eurozone country. Yet, for my work colleagues there appeared genuine shock that I had been away that long; some thought I was just a bit late back from lunch and were still busy working on many of the same familiar projects. One colleague was not even aware I had popped out for lunch! I am choosing to view this as an example of how much work takes over our life, rather than the other, less flattering interpretation …

Change is another difficult one to get your head around, especially if you only rely on the evidence of your eyes. The journey to work, including traffic jams, had not changed, and the office looked the same, give or take a few rounds of musical chairs. To the naked eye, everything looked the same. My office still had my 'to do' lists on the wall.

Plus ça change, plus c'est la même chose is all I can say …

* * *

Chemo can be fun on Fridays.

The day started predictably enough, with light following dark and kids sleeping in nicely after our thoroughly wonderful treat of tickets to Cirque du Soleil in a beautiful box courtesy of my brother's friends David and Kate. Things were not to remain normal for long, however, for chemo session number five …

'Has anyone got a bung for my oooji?' my chemo nurse asked the other chemo nurse who promptly and without the need for a translator provided the missing bung. I did not see where she inserted it. There followed an animated conversation with her colleague on how to hook me up to the drip from my portacath. I suffer a little deafness, but Beethoven himself would have been perfectly capable of hearing this conversation: 'I'm not very good at finding these portacaths, are you?' 'No, I don't like doing it, they move around too much. I tried her last time and after three attempts had to get Sam to have a go.' Undeterred by their lack of success, they made their way to me, brandishing needles, and, sure enough, had a good old game of Stick the Needle on the Donkey, although this donkey was playing hide-and-seek. Finally, on their third attempt, Sam was called and found the illusive portacath on her first attempt again. Champion.

In then came a shot of steroids called Dexamethasone, or Dexy's Midnight Runners as I call them. I hated them as much as I did the band, and while they did not sing *Come On Eileen* at the end of the evening, my legs did a passable impression of dodgy dancing and twitching all night long, so don't tell me that's a coincidence. An anti-sickness injection followed, and we were just about to keep to schedule when I noticed my name on the chemo was Brown, not Bown. Now, I have no problem with this as I have never been attached to surnames, but the chemo nurse was on the case: 'That dipstick boy doesn't know what he is doing.' Hmmm, not at all alarming then seeing as this dipstick boy is from the pharmacy that makes up the chemo, and I am pretty sure there is some strict science behind it. At least I hope he does not approach chemical recipes like I do food ones with a 'that looks about the right amount' mentality.

* * *

However, as I am getting used to life with cancer, nothing stays the same for long, and my newfound fun soon descended into the dreaded side effects.

I was not feeling in the least bit sorry for myself, but I just fancied documenting, while I remembered, the various inventive side effects of chemo and, in particular, a nasty little nerve drug called Oxaliplatin. On the days when my body cut me some slack and I felt normal again, I tried to 'love' this poxy Oxy in the hope that it was acting like a cold-blooded serial killer, showing no mercy as it hunted down the devious cancer cells. Sadly, it was not intelligent enough to weed out the bad guys from the good guys and just mowed down everything in its path, while I kept my fingers crossed that there were enough white blood cells left to keep the rest of my body going when Oxy had finished its latest two-week killing orgy.

But right when I was still struggling to throw off chemo round number five, I was not even on speaking terms with poxy Oxy or its sidekick, Capecitabine.

Chemo is cumulative, and I was beginning to really understand what that meant as the recovery period took a little longer each time and some of the side effects started to show signs of being a bit more permanent. I had read that the nerve damage brought about by Oxaliplatin could continue to muck you about for 18 months after treatment has finished.

I remember sitting in the oncologist's office before starting chemo and the Cheshire Cat telling me that no two cycles would be the same; as everyone reacted differently, there was no way of predicting who will get away with it and who will not. As it became clear that I was not going to 'get away with it', I was comforted with vague murmurings that it might mean (no one ever commits themselves to assurances) it was doing a better job on me and this could be interpreted as a positive sign. Thanks, Doc.

Let me regale you with my documented reaction to being nuked.

It is a three-hour process preceded by antiemetic sickness drugs that need an hour's headstart, followed by more anti-sickness drips and steroids before the Oxy infusion can be dripped in over two hours. Almost immediately I begin to feel my brain shutting down and the nausea starting to creep up on me as the last remnants of energy are sucked out. Before I leave hospital and step outside into the cold air, I must first mummify myself with scarf, hat and gloves as the smallest breeze freezes on my lips. (If I accidently breathe in cold air, it can cause my throat to go into spasm, which, having witnessed someone choking on my first chemo cycle, I never want to experience myself.) My fingers start tingling and any pressure or cold brings on extreme tingling sensations in hands and feet. This is called peripheral neuropathy. As it can be permanent, much care is needed to avoid cold, even to the point of taking something out of the fridge with gloves on! The most unpleasant feeling is the effect of the cold on my face as I feel my forehead, upper lip and nose freeze like a botched batch of Botox! On several occasions, my eyelids have dropped shut and have been unable to open in a kind of nerve spasm. My tongue swells and I am left with a nasty permanent taste in my mouth, only relieved temporarily by eating something strongly flavoured. It is strange how I can feel both nauseous and ravenous at the same time.

As Oxy continues its hunt around the body, I suffer first constipation and then the opposite. I have no idea whether this is caused by the Oxy or the steroids, but it all results in me turning into a jittery bundle of nerves unable to concentrate. By day 2, the heat comes and my face, hands and feet all feel like they are on fire. By day 3, I have horrid night sweats joined by the dreaded bone-and-skin aches,

*which seem to last for five or six days. Strangely enough, I
welcome this: although it feels like flu, with every pore in
my body aching, it is comforting to feel this lymph pain,
particularly strong around my face, neck and legs, as it
is proof to me that the chemo is circulating throughout
the lymph, which is jolly good news, considering that the
cancer had spread to my lymph and liver. At this stage, my
face is round and moonlike, although Mum says she likes
it as I look younger and smiley. I am glad to say it does
reduce in size again from about day 8 and starts to look
like the recognizable 'me'.*

    *I have got used to wearing sea-bands instead of
bracelets to counteract the nausea, and I am drinking
everything slightly warm, although I long for an ice lolly or
a really cold refreshing drink.*

However I still had some way to go before I could join the ranks
of post-chemo patients who have their brains washed into
remembering nothing less unpleasant than a little bout of flu!

*   *   *

Being a 'little bit under the weather' highlights the very essence
of being English. Our national character trait is to be self-
deprecating and crazily understated. We would rather chew
off our own tongue than be accused of the heinous crime of
boasting. Luckily, we disguise any whiff of a boast under the
cover of 'one-downmanship' that we show off when discussing anything remotely serious. But … it is still not enough to
shrug off our predicament in a dismissive manner; we must
also do it in a witty or amusing way.

How fortuitous for the English then to posses all the perfect characteristics to tackle the jaw-dropping embarrassment of having cancer or, worse still, talking to someone who has.

It is absolutely forbidden, for example, to answer the polite enquiry 'How are you?' with a 'Not very well, I have cancer'. This will be met with nervous coughs and raised eyebrows. You will have to be English yourself to appreciate how utterly discomforting those coughs can be. So a better answer perhaps would be 'Oh, not too bad, had a bit of the bowel and liver out, and my body looks like it has been knitted together by nanas, but mustn't grumble, had a few days off work!'

Humour is my favourite coping mechanism, and it strikes me that we are all at our best when we are laughing right in the face of adversity. So give me a dollop of irony, humour or mockery any day of the week, please.

One such example was a snippet of a conversation from a neighbour who stopped me in the street that morning: 'What I want to know is why are good people ill and dying, but when I turn on the television, murderers are still alive?'

Anyway, with Doctor Needles waiting patiently for his next fix of blood, I could not even graze the surface of this conundrum before rushing to have my second blood test in four days. Feel free to ponder now!

I was getting used to this double think – 'wanting' the chemo, but secretly pleased when it was delayed owing to my white blood count dropping, I presume like a feather, and labelling me neutropenic again.

Alas, I was provisionally booked in the following day for chemo round number six out of eight sessions in all, hoping that the painful G-CSF (granulocyte-colony stimulating factor) injection would work this time. My medical team had informed me that the muscle pain and flu-like symptoms I experienced for a week or so were a consequence of these bone marrow injections, so I was hoping they were doing something more useful than annoying me. The rest of the week was fully booked at the chemo ward, so I asked to be put on the waiting list just in case, which, Jenny remarked, was a mightily strange thing to put your name down for. She could understand if I was on the waiting list for a nice restaurant … but chemo, really?

All these delays meant the end date of my treatment was continually being pushed back, and the isolation was starting to do my head in. I thought about trying to volunteer at the local hospital, but they reminded me that being neutropenic and hanging around the factory where they grow germs was not recommended by people more intelligent than me.

* * *

Before cancer, I had never considered myself in any way a control freak and was happy to let chaos take over my life. But now I felt the need to write my numerous lists to stop me from losing the plot completely! However, once I began my new full-time occupation of visiting men and women in white suits, something strange happened: to my amazement, I tried to think ahead and build a plan encompassing occasional treats, visits and even possibly a bit of work. This had proved more wasteful and pointless than the British water industry.

So here's my advice to anyone trying to plan ahead: think of a number, add seven, triple it, take away the first number you thought … get the drift?

And so it was when my second attempt at chemo did not go according to plan that my blood played yet another of its hilarious practical tricks on everyone. It started with an early visit to hospital to extract more blood to see if my count had raised enough overnight to hit the minimum quota. Despite Mary Holloway, my brilliant Reiki therapist, encouraging me to drink more water, Dad making up even stronger Chinese herbs, Mum pumping me full of protein and top-needle nurse Sam hitting the portacath spot on first time, the neutrophils still said no.

If you can imagine getting all the little jobs out of the way that you know you will not feel up to over the next week or so and then adjusting the dimmer switch inside your head to 75 per cent off energy-saving levels, you will understand the frustration of being told, 'If you could just do that all again next week, we'll try again.' My plans for seeing Bear Grylls with my teenage son the following Saturday and possibly celebrating the end of treatment the following month were looking less and less likely.

So, I had another week off. It was sunny and the skies were blue, and after the initial disappointment, happiness descended. Superdad, however, was not impressed by this 'let's see how it goes' approach and set up another appointment with my acupuncturist to try moxibustion.

What, you might sensibly ask, is moxibustion? Well, let's just say my acupuncturist thought my blood was stagnant and, as all other methods were failing, we should try this. And 'this' was supposed to strengthen my blood, stimulate the flow of Qi and generally make me feel better. In traditional Chinese medicine, moxibustion is used when people are diagnosed as having a stagnant condition. You may also have heard of it being used to turn breech babies prior to childbirth!

After a lesson from my acupuncturist and armed with a packet of moxa sticks (made from the leaves of the herb *Artemisia argyi*, or Chinese mugwort), some diagrams showing the acupuncture points which relate to the movement and stimulation of blood and a set of instructions, we set off home to give it a go. There are points up my legs and my tummy which I could manage to reach myself, but Supermum, who has a steady hand, needed to be drafted in to reach the points on my back. Once lit, the moxa stick resembled a big fat cigar and you needed to hold it in place over the point or rotate it in circles and try not to burn the skin. The heat stimulated the acupuncture point and left me feeling completely calm and very, very tired. Something was happening, but I had no idea what.

* * *

While I was waiting for my white blood cells to recover from what was becoming their most stubborn sit-in, I decided to try another strategy to get things moving.

On a sunny weekend in March (yes, seriously, March!), I went to Brighton with my teenage son Joseph to shake things up a bit.

Used to conversing in complete sentences of only one word, it was a brilliant revelation to find that we could hold detailed and long conversations about all kinds of subject, from black holes to Bear Grylls: for example, 'How many bears can Bear Grylls grill if Bear Grylls could grill bears? Bear Grylls can grill one bear on his grill as he only has a one bear grill.' Or something like that.

Sadly, after the best weekend, we had to come back, for him to go to school and for me to go to the chemo ward. Would the 'Brighton' strategy work better than the numerous medical strategies to get the white blood cells moving? It appeared so …

With this being the longest ever delay to chemo, I had

felt quite normal for over a month and had almost forgotten what it felt like to be so ill, which proves my point about short memories where treatment is concerned. But I needed to get my head around the possibility of being nuked the following day as I attempted to get yet another blood test to see if my neutrophils were ready to rock.

I was totally caught out when my white blood cells stopped acting like French air traffic controllers and finally got back to work. Granted, they dragged their little white blood cell feet and needed to multiply in order to tempt them back into the chemo ward. But it goes to prove that you must never give up. A saying from Winston Churchill came to mind: 'If you are going through hell, keep going!' Life is anything but predictable, and it did me good to remember that faith and love were the key to getting through this.

As we descended back into winter that week, I could look forward to chemo swelling my body and face back up like an air bed over the following days. Plus the aversion to anything cold, which started immediately with my knife and fork causing my fingers to tingle. And even swallowing food was re-categorized as a dangerous sport once my throat went into spasms.

* * *

I do love gallows humour, but why do some people in the medical profession believe anyone facing the shock of a cancer diagnosis must be in complete denial and in urgent need of a nice little chat about death?

Personally, I would have thought this is the very time you could do with a bit of gentle brain reconditioning to build up your mental strength, but there appears a rush to unload both barrels on you faster than Quick Draw McGraw with the occasional book recommendation for your children on losing a parent lobbed in to lighten the mood.

Facing your demons is, in my opinion, a bogus concept that causes even more anxiety than the hard-working journalists from the *Daily Mail*.

Once upon a time I enjoyed the perverse pleasure to be had from a misery memoir, but these days I crave informed positivity and happy news even more than I crave the mute button on the Nickelodeon channel.

My own experience, which still stains my memory, was from a cancer charity who introduced itself with a motivational 'Hi, we are from the end of life and terminal care team'. Friends have also reported priceless gems such as 'I hear you want to talk about your death' to 'If you pay into a pension, I would not bother to continue if I were you'. Now should you manage to get over this punch in the head (possibly by holding your brain under a running hot water tap and scrubbing thoroughly for several months), there is amazing support, care and positivity out there and I cannot fault the dedication. It just seems a shame that we have to go through this ritual first, rather like an initiation into a street gang.

Surely, with the amount of evidence available on the effect of meditation, visualization and keeping a positive outlook, there should be more support focused here? I am sure I am not alone in calling for more guidance or training for the medical profession on giving life-changing news like this?

Anyway, I just about recovered my composure and was doing well thanks to all the support and medical attention I had received, and I hope the same can be said for any newcomers into the club. Roll on, chemo cycle number seven!

* ✳ *

The upside of my blood recovering meant that I went ahead with my penultimate chemo session as scheduled, and it all went super smoothly. I even got treated by a new nurse who put my steroids in by drip rather than by injection: amazing what passes for pleasure these days! And my good friend Jo did a changeover with Mum and turned up at lunchtime with liquorice toffees. Everything was going like clockwork … until I tried to leave and found the neuropathy and chemo fog had descended so fast that Jo resembled Usain Bolt as I tried to follow her to the car park. And this from a woman who broke both ankles and wrists last year, so I must have been hallucinating or the nice nurse had messed about with my wiring again.

Sure enough, sickness followed and my body began to emit its usual chemo glow lighting up the Chiltern Hills. You walk in to the sight of a miserable grey and rainy Buckinghamshire sky and leave a few hours later filled with chemicals – and hey, instant Maldives!

Chemo number seven was shaping up to be a nasty piece of work and roughing me up a bit too much. There appears no reason why one chemo cycle will be okay and another hell, but this session was the worst so far and appeared to stick me in neutral. Meanwhile, Dad, who was decorating my home, turned nurse and administered the bone marrow injections for me as my schedule had been thrown out so much that these now needed to happen on a Saturday when the hospital ward was shut.

Over the previous 12 days or so I seemed to have alarmingly slept IQ points out of my body. I would like to say that my dog sleeping on my bed had soaked them up, but he looked as vacant as I did still. My brain was as empty as a whistle, and I was stuck in a twilight world between being really sick and being really well and just needed to find the strength to jolt myself back into gear.

The one thing I did learn over those last couple of weeks was that there was no amount of telling myself I would feel fine again in a week or so which would convince the real me that I believed myself. Yes, I did have to reread that sentence a few times as well …

Of course, I could listen to countless people wiser than me informing me that I will start to feel normal soon, but knowing something and believing it are two very different states of mind.

The best advice is to be patient and remember that nothing stays the same for long. I could see that now as I was emerging from the fog and nausea. We all live in a constant state of flux, and hanging on to one state too long or worrying you are stuck with it is futile. I just needed to go with the flow and be ready for the next phase when it came along, as I now believe it will, and make the most of it when it arrives.

This is also valuable advice to any parent with teenagers. Admittedly, the units of time you measure these good moments might be nearer to attoseconds (the shortest time now measurable) rather than Olympiads (four-year cycles), but you get the point. Blinking during these periods is obviously not advisable. As they say: 'Change is inevitable. Unless you use a vending machine.'

But I now had something to look forward to on my third week of feeling good.

Table 8 at The Falcon in High Wycombe was fast becoming my favourite lunch spot. Glamorous it ain't. The inmates seem to think it most natural to drink pints at 11am, the fruit salads have as much fruit in them as beef tomatoes contain beef, and the wine comes out of taps, but it is a lot of laughs and I was in danger of returning again and again like a hand to a biscuit jar.

Kate, my new chemo friend, introduced me to this gem and shared the same aversion as I did for support groups, but we have luckily stumbled upon our own version which is a whole lot less earnest as we spent most of the time laughing like hyenas.

That particular week we dissected the personalities of the Siamese Cat and the Cheshire Cat, after discovering we shared the same double act. I was disappointed to discover that my memory of the Siamese Cat massaging my feet at the end of my bed was more likely to be a morphine moment confused with the post-surgery stockings rhythmically inflating and deflating on my legs.

Now, as I am sure everyone is aware, the medical profession is diligently trained to gasp silently to avoid alarming the patient, so naturally our oncologists' inability to dignify a question with an answer (if you don't count 'I wouldn't worry about that' or 'Let's wait and see') was viewed with narrow-eyed suspicion. However, after playing Oncologist Snap, we agreed that, in the case of the Cheshire Cat, this was less a case of deliberate suppression of bad news and more likely a reassuring positive personality quirk as I may have alluded to previously.

The biggest epiphany was the link between paper readership and cancer staging. As both of us had been *Guardian/ Observer* readers, we concluded that had we been lifelong subscribers to the *Daily Mail*, our cancer would not have reached T4! The *Mail*'s daily dose of cancer doom/cure stories would have seen us camping out in the waiting rooms of our doctors' surgeries demanding attention long before we eventually turned up, blissfully unaware that our colons were on their knees.

List of ways newspapers cover cancer

The *Daily Mail*: if you ain't got it yet, you will! Lock up your daughters, panic-buy supplies and get ready for the inevitable taking over our health service by the Romanians and Bulgarians.

The *Daily Telegraph*: make sure your private health insurance is top drawer, while maintaining a stiff upper lip. Hopefully, time to finish the round of golf first.

The Times: well, better to have cancer under the Tories – at least there are league tables and useful mortality-rate statistics.

The *Guardian*: keep looking on the positive side and if you are disposed to worry, then focus on Third World debt or the plight of the West Bank. Get over yourself!

---

* * *

'Rachel, Rachel, Rachel, what are you doing back here?' asked Dr Needles as if I were an Alzheimer's patient looking for somewhere nice to sit down.

When I sheepishly confessed I was hoping my blood had recovered enough from Friday to go ahead with my last chemo as planned, he tsk'd loudly and said I would have more luck stuffing an octopus with ADHD into my handbag or words to that effect.

Sadly, his predictions, as always, proved more accurate than the coalition government so far, and I was packed off home to put away my balloons and celebration cakes for another week.

Unfortunately, I was running out of things to do, but my lovely team saved me in the nick of time. I was very blessed to have enormous understanding and support from my work colleagues. Alex, my dear friend who also worked for me, acted like my own PPS (Parliamentary Private Secretary), and made sure that no whisper of stress reached my ears during the year and no doubt risked a coronary in the meantime. In cooperation with Sona, Anna, Shelley and Liz, they put together regular packs of titbits to keep me connected in a good way to the real world, but for my final session my entire team out-excelled themselves by sending me a chemo pack to jolly me over the line.

Here was my agenda for my final chemo courtesy of my team: Skittles for breakfast (on top of porridge, of course, don't be silly!); a spot of finger art printing; joining Danny Wallace in a cult; a nap; nun bowling; and looking for places to put apostrophes.

* * *

I am not a complete finisher. Up until now this finishing trait hadn't caused me too many problems, but I had no idea this personality 'defect' would be inherited by my body, which had enthusiastically decided to do anything other than finish building its immune system that week. However, it seemed to have enough time to make countless new grey hairs, layers of subcutaneous fatty tissue and excessive leg hairs.

As my final chemo was now long overdue, I (or, more accurately, my body) had decided against returning to the chemo ward this week, and after the recent shabby blood results, chemo was put off for another whole week.

My last husband, the father of my two children, has a Chinese wife (keep up!) who was training to be a nurse and who had started sending me lists of things to help with the cancer problem. This was much unexpected as prior to my insides rebelling we had never said more than two nods to each other. And now here she was raiding the NHS database for information to help my white blood count as well as suggestions from her native China on how to help.

It appears that, in China, it is commonplace for the oncologist to work hand in hand with a herbalist. Integrated medicine is the norm and you treat the mind as well as the body. There is a lot in my mind that, undoubtedly, would cause any Chinese practitioner to nod sagely and announce that I had much work to do to release my body from this disease (sic).

Chinese things I have taken up enthusiastically

1. *Acupuncture*. I have twice monthly, sometimes weekly, sessions and have found it helpful in restoring any tiny bits of energy and vitality. In particular, I have noticed the positive effect on my mind and a reduction in nausea and pain.

2. *Meditation and mindfulness*. I love this! After my last good night's sleep being sometime just before I hit puberty, I have learnt to sleep again! And I

➡️

---

can sometimes peek out from all this chemo fog. But, and this is most helpful, I can make decisions again as meditation helps me see things much more clearly.

3. *Chinese herbs*. Energy! Energy!! Energy!!! Very nourishing for the blood. I have no idea what they actually did, but I felt really good when I was on them (even if they did taste less pleasant than a bucket of cold sick). Be careful with these and check with your oncologist first. I did, and mine did the verbal equivalent of patting my head and smiling benevolently. I took this as a yes.

4. *Moxibustion*. Who knows what it actually does or how it works, but it was incredibly relaxing and I fell asleep immediately. It was without doubt the weirdest thing I tried during my treatment.

5. *Green tea*. I have grown to like it, and I now drink at least two cups a day. I also found out recently that, on top of the usual anti-cancer properties, it helps speed up metabolism. (And that is sorely needed after the effect of steroids, I can tell you!)

* * *

Faced with another week without chemo and temperatures ricocheting in true British style from 'coldest month' to 'hottest day' at speeds that would snap your neck, what else could I do than head towards Brighton for yet another treat courtesy of my Auntie Jane.

I was deeply touched by the many wonderful things my friends and family did for me. If you turned a blind eye to the hospital visits, it felt like a year-long birthday celebration.

And that week was no exception as we arrived in Brighton to be greeted by a glorious summer day: sun cream. *Check.* Sun hat. *Check.* Swimming suit. *Check.*

The sun was blazing, the clock said midday, a stray dog bounced along the beach: all we needed to complete the tradition were mad Englishmen …

'Last one to dip their toes in the sea gets a twisted ankle!' So off my Cousin Becca and I hobbled, choosing an obvious spot where the sea disguised an immediate vertical descent into the abyss.

Within seconds, my hat blew off into the sea, and given the choice of swimming with lanternfish, I stood paralyzed to the spot. A group of young men watched the drama unfolding and did a nanosecond calculation, but seeing two women of a certain age with their tops on decided they were otherwise engaged.

Not so my mum who, with reactions that would shame an antelope legging it from a cheetah, launched herself into the sea to save my hat, sacrificing my mobile phone to the waves in the process. One hat retrieved. One phone dead. And one mum a bit wet!

The week had been temporarily called the cake-and-wine diet and so, without further ado, we went for afternoon tea and demolished the lot. The following day, I completed the second leg of the challenge, sat in the sun and ate good food and drank good wine courtesy of my dear friend Di! Not a bad result. If that did not get the little white blood cells moving, they were simply ungrateful.

* * *

My white blood count had recovered enough to allow me to have my last chemo session, number eight!

While I was high on emotion, I gave a deep heartfelt thanks to my army of friends and family who had held me up when my knees or nerves buckled. To feel your love, to experience your kindness is the greatest gift cancer can give. So here's to you!

My family and friends who, when the going gets tough roll up their sleeves or trouser legs and jump in with me; people who have made me laugh and dried my tears; helped raise and comfort my children; made me endless cups of tea; walked with me when I needed to get out of the house; gave me wine when I could taste it; sent me weekly cards to keep the postman employed and me in stitches; talked sense into me when I needed it; reminded me of the good times past as well as those to come; sent millions of texts to let me know they are thinking of me and for not always expecting a reply; for loving me when I was at my most unlovable and boring; for listening to me when all I could think or talk about was cancer; for remembering to still ask me out as one of the gang even when it was unlikely that I could make it and, of course, for not taking no as an answer when offering help! For not treating me as a victim; for all your lovely smiles that hid fear or sadness; for coming to see me when I could not come to you; for keeping me entertained during the bitter winter and even colder spring months with delicious lunches; and for putting up with good grace my constant change of plans and last-minute cancellations.

And not forgetting my online family, those extraordinary courageous people who have pelted me with support and information and brighten my days when I need gentle stimulation or round-the-clock chat.

* * *

I was determined to be here again, racing for life. It felt neat and as if I was coming to the end of my treatment. I like things that are neat (despite being slovenly myself), birthdays that fall on even numbers, houses with even numbers, treatment all fitting neatly into a year – that sort of thing. So it was with enormous relief and a lump in my throat that I could risk the plug hole in the sky over High Wycombe being blocked long enough to allow some of my adorable friends and family to run the 5k Race for Life, a year after all this began!

It was drizzling and grey, but despite this I want to say a big thank you to Julie and Livvy Palmer, Tina North, Liz Waterson, Rachel Cramer, my niece Esme, aged 7 on her first run, and, of course, my lovely daughter Lois and my dear mum, for all running for CRUK and showing me such incredible support as well as raising well over £1,000 between them. I had planned to run it, but as I was still in the midst of my final chemo treatment, I was too poorly. However, I managed to stumble a few hundred yards over the finish line and to bag a medal to boot. But boy, did I suffer for it afterwards …

There's nothing like the sound of the starting horn and seeing hundreds of women each with individual stories of how cancer has touched them or their families to cause my throat to constrict and my breath to come in short staccato gasps. And this year was even more poignant remembering the same time last year when I ran the race with my daughter

and mum feeling poorly and just days away from being diagnosed with bowel cancer. So, quite seriously, here's to everyone
who has taken part, fundraised or donated. You make such a
difference and I, for one, am truly grateful.

* * *

Finally, I had to face the emotional roulette wheel that is called
a CT Scanner. After nearly a year of surgery and chemo, I could
now look forward to spinning around for the next few days in
limbo until it chucked me out on either the red or black.

I remember reading sensible advice about dealing with
'scanxiety' which, to put it simply, recommends distraction or
confrontation as a strategy for keeping your heart rate out of
the tachycardiac range.

Distraction was the strategy of choice, and, sure enough,
it presented itself, although not quite in the manner I had in
mind. Neutropenia had won again, and I had mysteriously
picked up a nasty little sick bug which visited me and resulted
in the Rennie Grove nurses sticking needles into my thighs
during the night to stop the sickness. I was no better in the
morning, so was told to take Nozanin, a strong sedative and
anti-sickness pill, during the day.

Here's where the challenge bit came in. I had to turn up in
the morning viewing the world through what seemed like a
film of bendy plastic, drink 700ml of white contrast dye and
then lie down in the scanner. Luckily, this was not the MRI
scanner that required you to train as an oyster diver in order
to hold your breath for eternity but a gentler one called a
CT. Despite a belly and armful of contrast dye, the Nozanin
tablets overpowered me: I nodded off and needed repeated
prodding and computerized voiceovers to get me to move.

Not the worst place I have fallen asleep, but I would not rush out and look for special offers on laterooms.com if I were you.

All these shenanigans left me feeling pretty numb and immobile. But I was encouraged by how well Lois was dealing with it all: when telling her about the CT scan that day, she interrupted and told me they now do magnetic nail varnish and then did a handstand! All is well.

* * *

So here I was facing the Siamese Cat, who had given me the cancer diagnosis and stamped a 'best before' date on me nearly a year ago. The same room, the same place. My mum, dad, brother and Jenny holding hands and breath.

And the news? I was in remission! But my goodness, didn't he make me work for it!

'Hello, how are you feeling?'

'Great … I hope. I just need to hear the results, please.'

'Oh, you had a CT scan, did you? When was that? How odd, my secretary did not warn me …'

Lots of rustling around on the desk and frantic logging in on the computer. 'Let me get the scan results up now.'

Oh dear, no, surely not. Where were the hidden cameras? We were going to have to do this live, anxiously watching every twitch on the Siamese Cat's face as he read the scan results out aloud for the first time in front of us.

After what seemed like an eternity discussing my bowel and liver surgeries and the fact that I had (unbeknown to me) another small cyst on my liver which he 'presumed' my liver surgeon knew about and which was not cancer, he said, 'Yes, this looks fine, you are NED (no evidence of disease) or NSR (no sign of recurrence).' And for extra emphasis, he added,

'Considering where we were a year ago and how aggressive it was, it's amazing we have got rid of it!'

I could have kissed him. He was grinning and said I looked really healthy. And believe me, this was a very good sign from the Siamese Cat who doesn't give good news lightly. His manner had changed, and he was all smiles and relaxed, with all the time in the world for me.

Joseph said that this day was the best of his life, and he could not stop hugging me. Lois was thoughtful and reflective and admitted to crying on the school bus with nerves. But she now sat so close to me that we could hardly breathe. I doubt I will ever know how deep this last year has affected them. Lois seemed to have taken it harder; maybe it was her age or maybe the fact that she tried so hard to keep everyone happy that she overlooked herself.

I had been given my life back and was deeply happy and thankful. Thankful to my two surgeons, my oncologist and the docs and nurses who have nursed me back to health. Thankful to my mum and dad and my brother who have loved me back to life. And thankful to my dearest friends and close family who never gave up hoping and had been by my side every day. And thankful to God for answering my prayers.

Now all I needed to do was to get the chemo out my system and start to feel normal again. The Siamese Cat said to expect for this to take about two months and up to a year. I took the last chemo tablets that night and chucked the rest of the tablets in the bin. They would be replaced by a diet of champagne!

NOW

YOUR PAST		YOUR FUTURE
MY PAST	THIS	MY FUTURE
YOUR PARENT'S PAST	MOMENT	YOUR PARENT'S FUTURE
YOUR CHILDREN'S PAST	CONTAINS	YOUR CHILDREN'S FUTURE
YOUR PARTNER'S PAST	ALL	YOUR PARTNER'S FUTURE
YOUR FRIEND'S PAST	MOMENTS	YOUR FRIEND'S FUTURE
YOUR WORKMATE'S PAST	C S LEWIS	YOUR WORKMATE'S FUTURE
YOUR BOSS'S PAST		YOUR BOSS'S FUTURE
YOUR BUILDER'S PAST		YOUR BUILDER'S FUTURE
YOUR CAT'S PAST		YOUR CAT'S FUTURE
YOUR EX-PARTNER'S PAST		YOUR EX-PARTNER'S FUTURE
YOUR OLD SCHOOL FRIEND'S PAST		YOUR OLD SCHOOL-FRIEND'S FUTURE
YOUR LOCAL TRAFFIC WARDEN'S PAST		YOUR LOCAL TRAFFIC WARDEN'S FUTURE
YOUR TWITTER FOLLOWER'S PAST		YOUR TWITTER FOLLOWER'S FUTURE

✳

What a difference a year makes!

When I woke up on the morning of 16 August 2012, my first thought was cancer. That was shocking as it sunk in that there must have been many days this last month when I had *not* given it a thought. And if you told me I would have felt like that a year ago, I simply would not have believed you.

Yes, it was a whole year to the day since I had been diagnosed with advanced cancer. I had planned to ignore the date as it was hardly an experience I wanted to relive like a treasured old cine film, but I could not help but say, 'What a difference a year makes!'

I was busy again, not sure doing what exactly, real life just got in the way. I would not have called it humdrum yet, and perhaps I never will again, but I was certainly rediscovering normality.

So what did this new stage of post-remission normality feel like?

Bonkers! I have ricocheted between numbness and the sort of emotional intensity that involves sideways tears and snot (sorry, mother). Some of you are probably nodding enthusiastically now.

I threw myself with unnecessary speed into a post-chemo party organized by my friend Julie, probably in an effort to convince myself that it was true, but most importantly, to thank the small army of wonderful people who had helped so selflessly. But I was lousy company, and despite having over 80 of my dearest friends and relatives over for the day and night, I wandered around almost mute with shock, strangely detached from the love and support all around me. This phase lasted 12 hours, and then the floodgates opened and I spent the next two days weeping at the hidden intensity of everything from utility bills to birds tweeting in the hedges.

A similar thing happened a couple of weeks afterwards when I spent time at a residential 'wellness' course at the Penny Brohn Cancer Centre in Bristol with my Cousin Rebecca for moral support. The first day was fine and dandy, but I had no warning I was to spend the entire second day with a box of soggy tissues screwed up in my hand and dissolving at the speed of a raindrop resting on a leaf or the smell of lavender on my hand. The emotional intensity was draining but necessary in coming to terms with what had happened and moving on, and I heartily recommend it to anyone. The people at Penny Brohn are wonderful and are doing incredibly worthwhile jobs. It was amazing how easy it was to get to sleep at night without the twin evils of caffeine and sugar (banned) propping me up like an old drunk in a whisky bar past closing time (although I am not sure another resident who confessed to smuggling in two litres of Coke and 30 years' supply of nicotine patches had quite the same experience).

But this reaction cannot just be me, surely? It must be a medical thing that your brain does to protect you from ever feeling that same sense of shock and disappointment again by a sort of elongated delayed response. I am going to call it 'dog looking for ball after you pretend to have thrown it' syndrome.

Or perhaps it is just the complete shell shock that accompanies the end of active treatment when you cannot quite believe you made it through. And all the pent-up anguish and trauma you went through finally hits – just when people expect you to be standing on tables or shouting from the rooftops!

Fittingly, though, this day was also the first occasion when I did not have a calendar appointment of future jollies to look forward to, so the few weeks or so before my return to work really were a test of my new humdrum. After a week of partying and chilling in Ibiza with the kids, Livvy, Jenny and Jade Jagger, followed by a couple of nights at an eco site in Dorset with torrential rain, mud and glimpses of sun, together with the unintentional setting fire to the tent, I was probably ready for it.

I have been reminded of my reason for living, and I don't ever intend to forget it. But for those of you still going through the worst of it, Nietzsche put it much better than me: *'He who has a why to live can endure any how.'* I certainly have that.

* * *

Cancer was my own Iraqi war. It was not a quick fight and home to glory. It was more of a long, messy war fighting an unseen terrorist with the long-term expectation that I would need to be on guard for years, until I knew my own body's fighters (the white blood cells) were able to take on the job themselves and man up to it. The date all being well is burnt into my consciousness – October 2016, five years after the last cancer had been taken out of my body. One of the last scuffles I was to go through before I could look forward to a long or even permanent respite was the reversal of my colostomy bag and the chance to put me back to pre-cancer engineering.

Before I got a new bum, I had a couple of CT scans. The first one was unscheduled and brought about by my thankfully overzealous surgeon, the Siamese Cat, who wanted to check (in his words) 'if the cancer had spread to my lungs or rib bones'. Well, who would miss a chance like that? The following seven days waiting for the results were incredibly unnerving, not to say uncomfortable, as he had also decided to throw in a mammogram for good measure.

Having got away with a clear on both fronts, he launched straight into my annual colonoscopy. The problem turned out to be costochondritis, an inflammation of the bits that join your ribs to your sternum. I think in my case it was caused by some over-energetic dancing …

Anyway, the thought of a colonoscopy was terrifying: not only the managing of the 'procedure' with a colostomy bag, but also erasing the shock of the last and only one. So I begged him to shovel as many sedatives into me as he could. To my relief, he obliged and administered a dose that would have rendered Michael Jackson catatonic. It was nice, though. And even nicer to hear that my bowel was still clear and in good enough working order for him to consider a reversal operation.

The clincher, though, was my six-month scan in December, the results of which also came back as 'no evidence of disease'. So I was delighted (under statement) to still be in remission and planning to get my body back.

But before I could again put on those paper knickers, tight socks and gaping back gown and sign the victim consent form, I had to endure a pre-op for my new bum.

It was a bit like going through check-in. My body was weighed instead of bags. Blood was extracted instead of cash. And questions were asked, loads and loads of questions, not to forget a serious amount of filing in forms. To distract myself, I decided to approach it as if I was ordering from an inflight menu and ticked enthusiastically:

No to CJD, Hepatitis or MRSA

Yes to ever having a serious illness

No to recreational drugs

Yes to not being shy on the legal ones

All fairly reassuring so far, you might say, until I came to one question which got me a little jittery: 'Is there anything else the surgeon or anaesthetist should know?'

Well, I can confess to having done a fair bit of swotting on abdominal surgery and watched entire episodes of *Holby City*, but I would not yet consider myself qualified to fill in any gaps in their knowledge. How flattering. Or worrying.

Anyway, all this activity was the precursor for a procedure called the Hartmann reversal. Procedure: an innocent enough word, you might say, but one which nonetheless takes on sinister connotations when mentioned in the same breath as hospital. But if you allow me to strip away the veil of medical mystery, what we had here, ladies and gentlemen, was a procedure for a new working bum.

And yes, I did get one for my birthday.

You may remember that the Siamese Cat kindly removed part of my recto-sigmoid colon, where the tumour was, capped the remaining rectal remnant inside me and rerouted the rest of my bowel to form a colostomy. He promised to try and locate the forgotten bit leading to my bum and join it back together with the other bit – with a staple gun. He planned to do this by keyhole surgery, but it would depend on how much scar tissue I had created. If he could not see what was going on, he would slice me open. That would be a bit of a pain as up until then bits of liver, gall bladder and bowel had all made their exits through tiny keyhole incisions.

After checking in into my hospital (I liked to think of it as mine; it was not much larger than an average house in Gerard Cross, and I knew all the staff and all 28 rooms), I was confronted by the usual test-of-nerve interview with my surgeon.

'Do you realize this is major surgery? I will attempt to do blah blah, but you must be aware of the risks of a leak that can happen when we try and rejoin the bowel. If this happens, you will suddenly feel very unwell about three or four days in and be rushed back into theatre, end up in intensive care with septicaemia and, of course another, bag. Do you want to pass go?'

'But the risks are very small,' I said motioning unsuccessfully with my eyes to my children who were in the hospital room waiting to see me off. By now, Joseph was shaking his head and sternly mouthing 'No, Mum' to me.

'Well …' followed by a prolonged shrug and sucking in of cheeks, 'about three per cent.'

Well, I'll be a monkey's uncle, that's okay then, what were we waiting for? Apparently a small delay for the Siamese Cat to sharpen his claws, peel both children off me – an historic moment as both were cuddling me so hard they had momentarily forgotten to argue over who had access to the most arms or legs – and we were off!

While prepping me for theatre, I happened to notice the trays of medical equipment and was particularly taken with

Guedel airways, less so with nasal airways. 'Where are we off to then?' I asked my Chinese anaesthetist. 'Where would you like to go?' he quipped. 'Mauritius?' I said, hopefully. 'Sounds good! I was born there, so let's go!' he said while administering a delicious cocktail.

I came round some four hours later and was wheeled back to my room, beginning to babble incoherently about Eric Bristow, the A405 and the Satsuma man. That's morphine for you!

Sixteen pumps of morphine later I was chucking up like a kennel full of sick dogs. So my precious pump had to be withdrawn, and I was forced to choose between pain control and sickness control. I opted for sickness control, somewhat unsuccessfully. After sampling every drug in the hospital and even one couriered in from another local hospital, my veins were collapsing faster than the price of Christmas puddings.

I will try to describe to you what the aftermath of a bowel reversal is like. Let's face it: if you have got this far in my book, you are not the squeamish type, are you? So I think we can move on.

The operation itself was a success. If you count success as stripping the bile from your stomach and throwing it up liberally over a six-day period and a total of four hours' sleep despite Temazepam and Tramadol (I am a professional pill popper), followed by weeks of uncontrollable diarrhoea and a numb *mons pubis*. Granted, it was only on the right-hand side but still an unexpected side effect. It almost made me want to rush out and get the right-hand side waxed, just 'cos I can. Sometimes you have to spot the bonuses and snap them up where you get the opportunity.

I was asked on what seemed an hourly basis if I had passed wind? How much? And whether it was loud or quiet! After three days of nothing, it was clear I was disappointing the medical staff, and the discomfort I was in was growing. I was told repeatedly that as soon as I passed wind or any motions, I would be relieved of this pressure. I worried that I was deliberately holding back on them. Finally, after three days and many walks around the ward with my drip later, it happened! And two days after that, the main event happened. I was warned it would be very loose as it passed through from my small bowel and they were not wrong. I immediately texted my parents: 'The eagle has landed.' (To borrow a phrase from my all-time hero, Lisa Lynch and creator of the legend that is *The C-Word*, no connection here.)

My text went viral, and my entire family appeared to be on 'poo' watch, asking for more information than I was used to supplying.

Eventually, on day 6, I was able to slowly introduce light food and get accustomed to the utter boredom of hospitals when you are feeling slightly well or at least well enough not to want to sleep through everything. By the weekend there were only two of us left in my new home and the other woman never left her room. So I wandered up and down the two corridors and earned multiple brownie points from the physiotherapist.

The good news was that the Siamese Cat was a miracle worker and had put me back together, mostly by keyhole, although I am going to have words as the exit wound was very much a letterbox or at least the keyhole for a set of keys that would not be out of place in a *Harry Potter* film.

After successfully managing to keep down soup (although I certainly would not recommend onions in your coleslaw), I checked out with a belly full of staples and some stickers to put over the old ones when they peeled off. So excited was I to be sleeping in my own bed again that I neglected to listen to any care instructions, or even read them for that matter, and luxuriated in a big deep bath full of Epsom salts as soon as I came home. This was silly.

The next morning I experienced a seepage and raw pain 'like someone has opened my scar and poured salt in it' I said completely oblivious to the irony of what I was saying. The next day I phoned the ward to check if the pain and seepage were normal, bearing in mind that I was supposed to be having my staples out the day afterwards and I was reluctant to let a fluffy cotton-wool ball near my wounded tummy, let alone a nurse holding a staple remover.

A short call to the ward later where my innocent explanation of bathing was met with a 'You've been getting it wet? You're not allowed to do that, it's an open wound'. And then the ominous 'I can't believe you don't know that. WHO CHECKED YOU OUT?' I spent the next ten minutes trying to reverse quickly out of the conversation and persuade the nurse that, of course, I remember now being told, and yes, it was my own fault.

One of the things you may notice is that your medical team does not always tell you exactly what you will experience. And that's an understatement! Hence any complaint will be met with a 'That's normal' response. Oh really? Would have been nice to know. My 'normal' was blood for two days/nights followed by constipation for four days followed by going 25 times a night reducing to about 8–10 times over a 24-hour period. However, I am sure if I had phoned my consultant and said, 'I have poo'd out ten sets of Liberty stationery and most of Staffordshire last night', he would have replied, 'That's completely normal. However, if you find yourself pooing out the South of France, please phone your doctor.'

If you are going through a bowel reversal op, here are some tips you may want to know.

Tips on going through a bowel reversal operation

1. Don't worry about your bowel restarting again. It can easily take a week, but it will restart. And when it comes, it will be very loose with blood, so don't be alarmed.
   (Until that point, though, you will feel quite uncomfortable and possibly sick. It will be a huge event met with cheering and clapping when you eventually pass wind!)

2. You will worry about the join and leak, but once you have passed wind and got past day 4, it is almost certainly good.

3. Don't eat any raw vegetables, fruit or onions in hospital. That's a bad move. Very small, often and bland is the key.

4. If in doubt, don't eat at all.

5. Expect the unexpected and learn to be patient.

6. It will take weeks to settle down.
   (To be honest, I was told it would 'never be the same again'.)

7. Exercise very gently regularly. You need to try and get mobile as soon as possible.

➔

---

8. It is a major surgery and therefore will be a major shock to your system.

(I was told the big internal muscles will take three weeks to knit, the external ones another three weeks, and all in all it will take three months to repair the tissues, so rest lots and don't lift anything heavier than a kettle.)

But to end on a more uplifting note, I was drawn to the practice of kintsukuroi which means to repair with gold. It is the art of repairing pottery with gold or silver lacquer and understanding that the piece is more beautiful for having been broken. My own repair was made with titanium staples – maybe not quite so beautiful, but, nonetheless, it is thought-provoking!

And to finish off the restoration project, I was finally deported ...

My 'power' portacath, or USB port, was removed. I knew that I was not out of the woods for years yet, but six months of clear CT scans were enough to make me want to get the last reminder of cancer apparatus out of my front body. And as my surgeon cheerfully reminded me, I could always have another one put back in if the cancer came back. Cracking news. But with a great big *caveat* that I still have private healthcare, because nuking you through a closed port straight into your jugular is classed as a luxury, naturally.

So, here's the drill for taking out a portacath. No sedation (more on that later). But lots of local anaesthetic which, I was warned, would feel like I was being stung by a bee. I put on a nice hat, was told to lie down and look to the right while I was covered in a sheet of plastic hooked over a drip stand, not unlike at an abattoir, I felt. A section was cut out, exposing my left chest and a stray boob.

There was quite a bit of cutting, shuffling and pulling around inside my chest to locate it and some rather disarming scraping noises. To avoid focusing on what was going on with my jugular, my mouth was unleashed, and I talked non-stop about all manner of nonsense. The procedure to remove the portacath took about half an hour during which time I learnt (or thought I learnt) that my surgeon stitched me up with pink cotton.

Any liquid I felt trickling down my chest was to be identified as follows: 'If it's warm, it's blood; if it's cold, it's pink.' My portacath was not 'stitched down' in position which I think explained the awful bother my chemo nurses had to keep the blighter still so they could stab it with one of their thick needles each time. And finally, my radiologist was a thoracic surgeon, and is also a part-time rock star – something I immediately looked up on YouTube. I mentioned that I was also on YouTube dressed as a banana giraffe to which he replied, 'Why doesn't that surprise me?'

The last words I heard him utter to his nurse while wiping sweat from his brow were: 'My goodness, we should have sedated this one after all. My ears are bleeding more than her wound.'

But I have my body back, finally …

A funny thing happened on the way to the shower a few days after the surgery to remove the portacath. I caught sight of my body in a full-length mirror. For the first time in over 18 months. I was suddenly aware that I had consciously avoided this moment since the shock of realizing that it had been letting me down all those months ago.

It was quite a moving experience. I did not see myself as someone who was scarred from three major ops, two minor ones and eight gruelling months of chemo but as a whole new person. I kept turning around and viewing myself from all angles, and I did not see the lumps and bumps and scars. I saw past all this and saw a strong body that had taken all that medical science could chuck at it and still bounce back for more. Stronger, I hope. No, I am not going all Californian on you, but I did feel more beautiful for it.

Yes, I have cared for it with pills and potions (supplied daily by Superdad), endless rounds of acupuncture and even exercise when I felt able to. Looking back, it was more like the care of someone who had suddenly been told to look after a friend's child. Of course, you feed it and keep it as safe and warm as you can. But you don't love it as your own. But at that moment, I did. Finally.

I am now ready to start treating, listening and learning to trust my body as mine again. I can stop thinking of my body as a selection of parts: the bowel bit belonging to one hospital (my extended home); the liver bit belonging to another hospital and consultant; and the chest and chemo bits to yet another hospital. No, my body is no longer the property of the medical profession. And to celebrate this epiphany, I took it shopping!

PART THREE

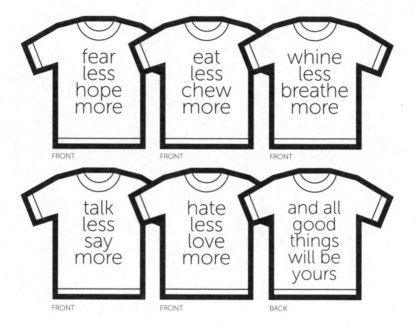

fear
less
hope
more

FRONT

eat
less
chew
more

FRONT

whine
less
breathe
more

FRONT

talk
less
say
more

FRONT

hate
less
love
more

FRONT

and all
good
things
will be
yours

BACK

Swedish proverb

CHAPTER FIFTEEN

✳

The new normal

So what is the new normal?

At times, I am feeling guilty. Guilty for surviving when others who were diagnosed after me, and who were even younger than I, have died. Guilty for still going on about the cancer long after the drama of treatment has finished. And guilty for all the trouble and worry I put my loved ones through.

At times, I am feeling scared. Although life is fun again, after cancer, it doesn't take much to flip back into 'rabbit in headlights' mode.

I also seem to be feeling more emotional occasionally. I call it a faulty emotional volume button in my head. A bit like those hearing aids that are given out to annoy OAPs! I had no idea when the volume would suddenly go all high-pitched. But I was certainly aware I was becoming hypersensitive to most things, physically and emotionally.

The new normal involves having to take a strong hold on my finances. Living for the moment is expensive. 'Never spend tomorrow when you can buy it today' is utterly enjoyable, but financially disastrous! My life expectancy may be less clear, but my wardrobe and makeup collection have gone from strength to strength ... as has my 'life's little luxuries' budget.

I am learning to do 'whatever it takes'. A close friend who recently experienced loss advised me that she had to pull herself together because 'people don't want to be around you if you are permanently giving off negative vibes'. She attacked this challenge with predictable managerial control, and has a repeat prescription set up at the doctor's ready to call on. It provides Citalopram (an antidepressant), Zopiclone (sleeping pills) and Co-codamol (pain relief) when she feels she needs a bit of rescuing. She keeps this quiet, but it has given her the tools to be herself and to fully engage with life again.

I am dwelling on my achievements to date, not my possible failures in future. I have produced and raised two wonderful kids, attracted some fantastic friends, secured a jolly good job, seen lots of the world and experienced real intellectual and physical pleasure. What I can or cannot do in the future is too abstract and disarming to dwell on today (or any other).

Sorry, Mum and Dad, but I am enjoying taking a few more risks than before. Nothing is as Herculean as it once felt. You get used to feeling neat high-concentration euphoria (after clear scans) which can result in the odd flirtation with changing my life dramatically. I had difficulty dealing with the mundane again at first and rebelled at any chance to make me conform.

The new normal also involved learning to deal with the clammy fear of the cancer reoccurring. I found I had a serious mistrust of my body now that we were alone again and needed repeated confirmations that things were really okay. I also felt pretty angry about conversations that went 'That's so amazing, you are cured. Must feel incredible now it's all over'. Guaranteed to throw me into instant irritation. Yes, of course, I am happy that it is over, but I am dealing with the constant and very real fear that it will come back.

I am sure my family must have thought my end of treatment meant the start of their new normality, too, and a chance to have a well-earned holiday. I know they had put their own lives on hold since the very first second, and it was time for them to go home and reclaim their house and lives. But we were forgetting: *Mi casa es su casa!*

My house was not looking too shabby as Superdad had been around daily to do all those little 'Botox' jobs that need doing in a house of a certain age. And to top that, there was always a fire roaring so that it was warm and welcoming. My fridge was full of delicious organic food (courtesy of Superdad and Supermum's weekly small-farm organic orders), and the kids had become accustomed to living like a Mediterranean family, with everyone eating and living in the same house. No one wanted the status quo to change.

How do you suddenly stop being responsible for the fire, food, juice, shopping, odd jobs and general children duties? Dad, who relishes any chance to be in control, had to learn to ease up on all these auditing and responsible jobs and was urged (nay, targeted) by Mum to try and get in and out of my house in under two hours! This caused some stress as Mum would try to cut down on the multiple rechecks before Dad considered it 'safe' to leave. Mum: 'You are just double-checking something you have already checked; it's not necessary.' Dad would flinch and reply: 'I just need to look at the fire again. Have you checked the back door?' A typical conversation would continue:

'Don't start counting cutlery like you do when you're stressed!' says Supermum.

'What did you say?'

'Nothing, dear.'

'Someone can see the knives and stab you. It could happen. It *does* happen …' (Dad would not live with a knife block in his house.)

'There's some grass on the floor.'

'Yes, dear, I can see.'

'You have somehow managed to get it all over the kitchen. Dear, oh dear.'

'Yes, you have checked the door. You don't need to repeat it three times.' And on, and on …

But you will be relieved to hear we have hit a compromise. Dad will bring around a daily (or if I can get away with it, every other day) juice as well as the delicious wheatgrass. You might conclude this is a simple arrangement, but it involves organic produce being cut up and washed, a 'special' machine to juice this concoction which, of course, needs assembling, disassembling and washing and each component needs drying individually and very carefully.

At some stage, your family has to stop wrapping you in bubble wrap, cooking, shopping and cleaning for you. Naturally, you want them not to pay as much attention the minute you mention you are tired or cannot sleep. Everyone who has been on this cancer merry-go-round with you needs to get back to a new normal.

* * *

I have come to the conclusion that cancer is a very British disease. But I cannot keep going around saying 'sorry' daily. Anymore than I can go around saying 'Yes, I'm feeling so high I could lick the surface of the moon' (just in case the mere deviation from an unbearably upbeat tone signals potential doom), but there must be another way of dealing with this post-remission business. One that doesn't send people reaching for their sick buckets or the off switch.

Now, the next bit is probably the hardest bit to write as I can almost hear the pages closing as you no doubt think, 'Boring, she's in remission, not much drama here, then.' And you'd be right. Drama is limited. But there is still humour and loads to learn. I am more than aware that bad news sells, and well, it is just that much harder to tell a story that ends well. Yes, once it was clear I was not going to join the grim reaper in a spot of gardening, my blog hits dropped fast. But I am assuming if you are reading this far, you may have a vested interest in cancer and stick with me a little longer! Of course, you can keep popping back to my blog to check I am still alive. In which case, thank you, it will coincide with a dramatic increase of my web traffic and book sales. I remember being terrified when I first got diagnosed and starting reading cancer memoirs, got emotionally attached and then took a massive dive when I found the author had since died. I seriously considered all books should be re-issued with a 'Now dead' stamp on them to avoid disappointment.

So bear with me and I promise not to lapse into self-help speak or evangelical fervour, but throw some light on some good, honest truths. That way, you cannot say you were not warned if you stumble into these territories unarmed and make the classic boo-boo of saying 'You'll be fine, I've no idea what you're upset about, you should be on cloud nine'. And then swiftly move to another subject and leave with a dead leg, bruised cheek or more than likely, 'cos we're British, a polite cold shoulder and a lifelong grudge!

* * *

I was having a conversation with myself the other day where my old brain was trying to reprimand my new brain for its lack or organization and tidiness. It was lamenting the state of the living room that resembled a snow storm in a sweet shop, with the fluffy white inside of the dog's bed mixing with the daughter's hundred and thousands bits from an ongoing cooking incident. As well as the garden looking like a graveyard, with the half-finished nuclear bunker, being dug by my son, vomiting up six square feet of mud against my back fence.

When I suddenly stopped short.

I came to such an abrupt halt that I felt my new brain piling straight into my old brain; the bit where self-control resides, also referred to as the fronto-median cortex. This can only mean that further episodes of impulsiveness are likely.

Anyway, I digress.

Since being in remission and resuming normality, I feel I need to remind myself how I felt when buying products from the long-life section in supermarkets seemed like a shocking waste. Reminding ourselves of what is important and what is not while we still have a life is as essential as breathing.

Life's too short ...

1. Not to buy what you love because you don't know where you will wear it.

2. To turn the heating thermostat down when you are cold.
(Yes, I know all you pre-1950s babies had to chip ice off your undies and also wee outside.)

3. To pretend to be a UK size 12 when everyone knows you are really a 14 on a good day.

4. Not to let the dog sit on the sofa/bed/car seat.

5. To stick with the same haircut all your life.

6. To pretend to like anything just to impress someone.

7. To get up early on your day off.

8. To buy cheap transparent adhesive tape.
(You know the type that tears lengthways instead of widthways.)

9. To over-plan. Whoever really answers the 'Where do you see yourself in five years?' question with any honesty?

10. To think of a number ten just to round things off neatly.

→

> ### ... and now for some slightly more serious stuff:
>
> 1. Not to take a day off to go to your doctor when you have a niggling fear that things are not quite right or let embarrassment get in the way once you do.
>
> 2. To hold on to anger or grudges, especially with family and friends.
>
> 3. To lose sight of what is important to you in life. Ever.
>
> 4. To not say what you mean, because you are scared people will like you less.
>
> 5. To wallow in self-pity.
>
> 6. To not tell people you love them.

* * *

I said at the outset that I wanted to live long enough to teach my children resilience. So naturally you are going to want to know how I am doing.

The dictionary definition of resilience seems to be something that can return to its original shape after being deformed. Rubber, for example. Which means my liver is probably resilient having regrown to its original shape, but my bowel does not have the same powers and is therefore a failure in the resilience stakes.

But to me, it means being able cope with whatever is thrown at you and not lose yourself or give in. I want Joseph

and Lois to be able to deal with painful emotions and disappointments and turn all that pent-up anger or sadness into
something useful.

I am super resilient. But in my effort to downplay everything, I think I may have played the children resilience challenge a bit wrong. I read a piece about resilience, especially
aimed at the anxious child, in the *Guardian*. And let's face it,
seeing your mum go through what I have been through would
be enough to make the most sanguine child anxious.

To paraphrase the *Guardian*, I need to stop reassuring
them and telling them they will be fine or that there is nothing
to worry about. I am supposed to be asking open questions to
help them figure it out and reassure themselves. I tried this
today with the teenage boy: 'Joe, are you happy with the work
you've put in for your food tech homework?' 'What work? You
did it.' Okay, so that may not be the answer I was looking for,
but if I do this often enough, it should become second nature
allegedly.

The next test for us is to stop giving them the answers. I
have to teach them to manage their time better by making lists
(maybe there is something in this after all) and prompt them
into chunking down their tasks into manageable bits. I tried
this again with Joseph: 'Shall we sit down together and think
of three ways to make learning maths easier for you?' 'Pfff … I
HATE maths. MUM, I'm watching this (insert anything more
preferable to maths; the list is inexhaustible).'

The next one I like – the worst-case scenario. Thinking
through the worst that can happen is second nature to me,
and I do quote it often enough and am hoping it will ring
bells: 'If you go into school with your new haircut on Monday,
what's the worst that can happen?' 'I'll die. Mum, seriously you
have no idea. Your advice is useless!'

Furthermore nerves are good. They are a sign you are excited, and this is good energy to help you focus more. Do they believe me? I also need to teach them to breathe in slowly doing the 7–11 technique: breathe in counting to 7 and out counting to 11. Lois tried this during her gymnastic competition over the weekend. She did not get a medal and so also declared my advice 'useless'.

Joe is physically very resilient. This year, he has spent many nights sleeping outside in his tower that he built in our garden in temperatures below freezing. He has also equipped each member of our family with their own survival packs and detailed instructions on what to do if our little village of Holmer Green ever becomes a threat that needs extinguishing.

However, I am left in no doubt that he could survive a good deal longer than me if the luxuries of life were suddenly removed and we found ourselves camping (again!).

But emotionally – nah, that's a totally different matter. This is still very much a 'work in progress'. He still treats me as if I am fragile; every journey is accompanied by 'BE CAREFUL, MUM, DRIVE CAREFULLY. PROMISE!' Every evening out is accompanied by a phone call: 'Where are you, Mum? When are you coming back? You've been out late. You're NOT drinking, are you?' I realize I have turned my son into my dad. This was not on the agenda.

Whereas Lois is more emotionally resilient, but is a little more fragile on the physical side. Here's a recent example of her resilience. She had been 'going out' with her boyfriend; it was a union that his mum and I very much approved of (and even that did not deter her) for six months, and I worried every week that this would be the week it would end. How would she cope?

She coped as naturally as any 12-year-old would. Buckets of tears. Hours on the phone and Facebook to friends followed by cuddles and hot chocolate and then finally topped off by ... a jelly bath with her best friend Livvy! The pair of them were literally up to their necks in a bath that had solidified into jelly.

So, in every sense of the word, she is a bouncer. But physically I worry more; there are many worries about 'tummy problems' and trips to doctors and hospitals to investigate. How will I know when to push for answers or when to soothe as it may be a reaction to my illness? And who would blame her?

I think that, like me, they are experiencing fear as a delayed reaction. In hindsight, we realized we were all afraid.

Ultimately, though, I want them to be resilient enough for me, too.

My top tips for Lois

1. Do **not** drive a car until you are at least 20. And do **not** get into a car with a boy, until he has lost his boy racer stripes. At least five years' wait, please.

2. Keep on being an individual.

3. Do not drink alcopops. If you have to drink spirits, make sure you buy more rounds (it is only money), just drink the mixers – avoid peer pressure. No one will know (I have been doing it for years ...).

➡

4. Never compare yourself to other girls who cannot hold an Olympic-sized torch to you.

5. Pay attention! To everything: cars, roads, men, all modern dangers ... Pointless me telling you to listen more and speak less as we are so alike and I am still learning, but try. Please!

6. Enjoy the journey as much as the destination. It is not all about the badge you get at the end.

7. Do not ever settle for a boy who is not worthy of you. Ever.

8. Oh, and keep on laughing until you cry.

My top tips for Joseph

1. Do not get into any car with more than one boy or girl in it.

2. Remember the cup-of-water thing I taught you: don't carry it around all day, put it down.

3. You share half of Lois's genes, so be nice to her, please!

4. You are very, very funny and clever. And unique. I just wished you would believe it. You will one day, but think of all the time you will have wasted by then.

5. Don't worry. Worry will not stop the bad stuff happening, but it will ruin the good days in the meantime.

➡

6. Please keep at something longer than it takes for the guarantee to wear off. There are not many short cuts in life.

7. Remember that mobile phones are useful as is all communication.

8. Please smile (not the sideways one that looks suspicious. The big one!) and answer people when they speak to you. It is surprisingly effective.

* * *

I often get asked this question, so I will attempt to answer it as honestly as I can. Speaking as someone whose default setting has always been jammed stuck (no doubt with chewing gum) on fast forward, the year or so of enforced rest has allowed my poor overtaxed neurons to light up what is important and what I have no need to meddle with anymore. And while I certainly would not recommend 'excess cell mutation' as a sabbatical of choice, it sure does wonders for your sense of perspective. So here is what I have learnt and want to hang on to.

The view from the bridge

1. *Worrying will not add a single hour to your life.*

2. *You are much stronger than you think. Congratulations!* You will not know this until you are tested. But trust me on this one.

➡

3. *Nothing stays the same forever; just hang on tight when it gets stormy.*

Everything passes eventually, good or bad. It felt like I was in a maze and could not see my way out, but once I was shown the route, it got easier. Of course, I could not remember the way out the next time I was in ... but I tried to remind myself that I did get out last time, and I will do the same again, after I have gone down a few pointless avenues.

4. *Life is a precious and unpredictable gift, so live your life, not someone else's.*

5. *Your family will be your lifeline.*

Like John Diamond, I did not need cancer to remind me how much I loved my family and how much they love me, but there is no doubt it has brought us together much closer and taught us to say how much we love each other while we can. It has taught me the meaning of true, uncomplaining selfishness. I don't know who has been getting all the normal moans and groans of life, but it has certainly not been me! Don't ever stop appreciating your family.

6. *I have learnt the real meaning of friendship.*

People are infinitely more loving, kind and supportive than you believe (we Brits just need an excuse to open up and show it sometimes). I have learnt

➡

the value and meaning of true friendship. Those
wonderful individuals who have been by my side
from the beginning, through the long boring winter
months, and who are still here at the end of my
treatment. Cancer feels a bit like bereavement:
there are many of us who are good when we hear
the news, offer support and comfort and remember
the anniversary each year, but to be there during
those silent months when most people have left you
alone is the sign of true friendship. I have been truly
blessed with such individuals. You know who you
are. I hope I can remember this and repay a fraction
of this love when the time comes. I have never
felt so loved. Keep in touch with those who have
touched you in whatever way you can.

7. *You cannot control cancer, but you can control your
own medical records.*

Don't rely on your doctors alone. Keep a copy of your
records. Keep your diary appointments, chase up
and never expect people to get back to you. Ask for
second opinions if you are unhappy with a response.
And educate yourself so that you are not fobbed off.
Remember: you need to be a type A personality!

8. *You cannot control cancer, but you can control your
own mind.*

What you read in the first few weeks is crucial. So fix

➡

your mind early on. I searched out funny, positive stories and avoided being dragged down by other people's sad stories. There are days when you can cope with looking over the precipice, and there are days when you must not look any further down than the kerb.

9. *Take one day and sometimes one hour at a time.*

Cancer is unpredictable. Things can change for the better as well as for the worst. I have lost count of the number of people who were told they were inoperable at the beginning, then went on to have chemo or radiotherapy and were subsequently operated on. As a good friend of mine told me at the beginning: 'They are treating you. That's what you need to focus on.' Even if they do not promise a cure, treatment is improving every month; so don't ever give up hope.

10. *Power down sometimes and give yourself permission to just stop and fuss less.*

I was my own worst enemy. I felt that I needed to keep going and was letting everyone down if I stopped. It took me many lessons, painfully repeated, to realize that I did not need to be in control of everything. I just needed to know how to react.

➡

11. *I am not indestructible. I am not guaranteed 30 more years, three more years or three more minutes ...*

Each and every day is a gift, so make the most of it. Wake up! You are incredibly lucky to be alive. Sometimes it takes a *big* shake-up to realize what is important to you and what life is all about, and that's okay.

12. *Enjoy and love what you have while you have it.*

Of course, I am not talking about material stuff. No, what I mean is that each day is a bonus, and you should treat it that way. Each person you choose to have in your life is a blessing. Learn and spend time with them, and enjoy their company, because they may not always be there. I cannot put it more simply than be thankful for your life, live it and love it. I have never wanted to live so much in my life. I feel more than I have ever done before, and nothing is taken for granted anymore.

13. *Cancer can happen to anyone; it is random and complicated.*

Cancer is random. It is a thousand times more random than Paula Hamilton in *Celebrity Big Brother*. It is not personal. I have met some of the nicest, most generous, caring people sitting in the chemo chair beside me. Cancer does not care about race or sex, how fat or thin you are, or how good of

→

a person you may be. It often strikes silently and without much warning. There is no way to prepare for it. Once you are diagnosed, you are stuck dealing with something that most people have just had passing thoughts about and then decided not to think about because 'it's not going to happen to me'. Claims of cures are often simplistic at best. However, I am a big believer in helping your own body fight cancer and the importance of supporting your own immune system to do this.

14. *People have the best of intentions and truly want to help and be supportive.*

    Of course, most people will fumble in trying to say the right thing, but on the whole, I have been overwhelmed by how fundamentally caring and supportive people are. I am bombarded by good will. I should not have cancer, and we all know a lot of people who should not have had to suffer through it either. It is a tough pill to swallow, but the sooner you realize that you cannot control your diagnosis but only the way you *handle* it, you will be able to feel more in control of the disease. You will also notice some of the small 'gifts' that this disease provides, like the 'gift of perspective' – which is one I personally would never want to have taken away.

15. *It is not just about you!*

    Your nearest and dearest are watching you go through this and need a shoulder to cry on, too.

    ➡

Make sure they get time off and plenty of support. They will be going through the same reactions as you, sometimes a little delayed, but it will hit and you have to be there for them when this happens. The Macmillan 'Not alone' campaign in 2013 dramatized this beautifully: 'Today 889 people will be hit with the news they have cancer; then it will hit everyone who loves them.' How poignant and true.

* * *

I awoke to news that I may have a stiff upper lip. That may not sound fatal to you ... but are the UK's poor cancer survival statistics down to a humungous Victorian hangover or do we need to look a bit deeper than this stereotype?

I am not an anthropologist, but I would suggest we could do with some serious observations of our macho culture, our 'importance of not being earnest' culture (guilty, M'lud) as well as our 'too busy' culture before we jump to conclusions.

Looking at this from the perspective of bowel cancer (über-embarrassing) and my own experience, I am not exaggerating when I say that 100 per cent of all younger patients I have come to know over the last couple of years claim GPs 'shrugging off' their symptoms or lazy labelling was the norm. The cost of this is shocking and tragic because so many young families are living with the realization that they may not see their children grow up, or perhaps ever be parents themselves.

So yes, how many times do you get knocked back before you start to feel embarrassed about wasting your GP's time? I certainly did not start out as being embarrassed. But factor in continued rejection when you talk about your bottom and I challenge anyone not to get embarrassed! In fact, the first time I heard the 'poo' word mentioned, it was from my surgeon who threw around 'poo' liberally in every sentence without a shred of awkwardness.

But is there also a story around our macho culture and our long working hours causing reluctance to visit our docs? I would rather chew off my own tongue than be described as a hypochondriac, so my colon was practically on its knees before I sheepishly went back again for a third time.

This is a recipe for disaster! Busy, sometimes poorly trained doctors and a patient with a stiff upper lip!

So how can we remedy this?

1. *Greater awareness of symptoms of bowel cancer*: especially its effect on younger patients (2,000 diagnosed each year, and I am willing to bet, we might be diagnosed at a more advanced stage than the norm).

2. *A touch of 'Scandinavian' lip*: come on, you can say it, 'poo'.

3. *We need GPs to take us seriously*: they should help us articulate/prompt us/question us. In my experience, it was a one-way street. If we are sitting in front of you, chances are it took a Herculean effort to get there, so interrogate us!

4. *Get serious about your symptoms*: research and educate yourself.

Oh, and can someone please do research on how many times a patient visits their GP over, say, a 12-month period before finally being diagnosed. I bet *that* would make interesting reading!

* * *

Initially, all I wanted to be was clear. But it took a long period of adjustment coming to terms and trying to slip back into life. How do you adjust? How do you stop feeling like an outsider? There were days when I had difficulty relating to conversations. I had no idea on how to shut the door where the cancer memories lived. The answer is: you don't. You will always have a special connection to people who have gone through it which is difficult to break.

One of the things that has been bothering me is: do I really know what people now think of me? Are people being true with me or are they hiding part of their inner life for fear of sounding shallow? A typical conversation would go: 'I have just had XYZ (insert illness, personal catastrophe or choice in here), but of course it's nothing like you have just gone through.'

And what do people really mean? I met some friends of my brother at a party recently, and when I was introduced as 'David's sister', I may have been a bit paranoid, but a moment's hesitation was followed by 'Oh … how nice to meet you. How are you?' I was confused.

Did this 'How are you?' mean to expect nothing more than the customary 'I'm fine' response and to move on? Or was it a 'How *are* you?' In other words, are you about to cop it? Am I only now hearing the subtitles of life? And how do I avoid this?

I have tried shock treatments: 'Your good deed of the day is to take a cancer patient (me) out and shock me back into the land of the living with good old-fashioned gossip.' Failed.

I have tried denial: 'Never better, thanks. Hardly ever think about it, to be honest.' But I could not help adding in a dollop of sarcasm: 'Nothing more than a scratch, really' – which I think fails spectacularly.

I have tried distraction: 'So, how are *you*? I won't let you leave until you tell me every last bit of news.' This was slightly more successful, and this tactic might well help those people I know, or have known, for ages. But what about those I meet for the first time since? When do you 'drop' it into the conversation? Too early and you appear needy. Too late and you might be accused of hiding a major part of yourself and not trusting the person. These rules change depending on whether it is work related, family related or date related.

I had been back at work a week and I had an appointment to see the new CEO (who had been appointed recently in my absence). I found myself over-preparing for this meeting. I had to convince him not only of my abilities but also of my longevity! So I naturally consulted my 12-year-old daughter for fashion and makeup advice. Not so much of a 'How to look good naked' challenge but a 'How to look healthy' one. I banked sleep. I wore a dress that was aiming for a look somewhere in between professional and Cameron Diaz healthy. I added lip gloss and highlighter on my cheeks. A spot of hair dye on the grey hairs and I ran up the three flights of stairs beforehand to achieve that healthy glow.

I was ready. Or so I thought. First question: 'So what do you think is the best structure for your team?' No awkward health-related questions. Just dived straight in. I must look viable!

The second test was men. Hmmm. A funny old invention, men. I genuinely had no desire nor felt ready for a relationship. I did not want to be anyone's everything. Apart from my children's, of course. (Mother/Father, if you are reading this, don't pass out, I am only half serious.) But, and I am taking this as a sign that I am feeling much better, occasionally I thought it would be reasonably bearable to go on the odd date or two (as long as the chap in question had his own home, job and life and was not keen on taking over mine anytime soon). How do you go about this? There is the sensible way and there is the Rachel way. What do you think I chose?

The scene of crime was a music venue, packed shoulder to shoulder with men of a similar certain age. So far, so interesting. 'Hello, down there!' Beg your pardon? I looked up to see a tall chap who did not look half bad, even in this light. Surely he was not addressing me? But it looked as if he wanted to continue the conversation. I raised myself up to my tiptoes and tried to shout above the music into his ears which were at least a foot above my own. After a long exchange of pleasantries I learnt that he was divorced (good; I don't mean 'good', but at my age, if they have never had a long-term relationship/ marriage, it is not looking 'good' either), father of two children (good), sole carer as his wife had chosen career over kids (oh no, that's a killer line, now I think I am melting), runs his own gardening business (more good, nice and grounded), had his own house (even better), was very busy as he had his kids three weeks out of four (excellent), lived half an hour away (perfect), was a few years younger than me (not tried that before), had a very interesting life and friends (sinking fast) … and what was weird was that he was appearing to be chasing me! The chase continued for an intense week. It was long enough to remind me that I am still attracted to doing everything at dizzying speeds and, despite my newfound wisdom and wish list, realized I still did not do semi-detached very well.

Unfortunately, there came a time when I judged it just about right to lob in the 'cancer' bit. I had got myself trapped down a few conversational cul-de-sacs where I was having difficulty explaining what I was doing 'not at work' or why I was 'writing a book'.

I played it down. I emphasized that I was healthy now and

going back to work shortly. I did not even mention poo! But I could already see the flirtation fizzling out like a duff firework. Despite assurances that it did not 'freak him out', the lack of questions and the speed in which he left was enough of a sign that this was perhaps the last I would see of him. And it turned out to be the last I heard from him as well. He had calculated his return on his emotional investment and obviously found it wanting.

The bit that threw me the most from this fanciful distraction was not just the clear rejection for not ticking his 'survival of the fittest' box but the unsettling few weeks afterwards having been shown another life which I quite liked the look of. And I found my previous satisfaction with my single life being tested a bit over the next few weeks. For this reason alone, I was fuming.

Yes, I hear you shout collectively, 'You haven't met the right bloke yet.' You may be right. It turns out I got conned by a cad. *I* know that. *You* know that, but still …

For this reason, I like to hang out with people from time to time who have been through the same as it is the only time we can be truly honest with each other and even share some dark humour. Liz, a friend who shares the same surgeries, prognosis and surgeons as I do, has a wicked streak and has been known to ask in company: 'How are you? Still alive or have you had a relapse yet?' or if I sit down awkwardly: 'Ouch … Oh, you poor thing, are you sure it's not spread to your pancreas?' Over lunch at our darling mutual friend Di's house when Di might ask me something about the cancer, Liz would pipe in: 'Oh? Did you really have cancer? I'm sure it was only a bad cold?' What pleasure we have in throwing death around without having to deal with the sensitivities of the non-ill. Our bimonthly get-togethers were better than any support group. Di's lunches were legendary; if they broke up before 4am, it was considered lightweight.

Anyway, what I have learnt is talking about cancer may well be scary, but *not* talking about it is even scarier!

For my friends, family and work colleagues who went through cancer with me, I feel we have a shared experience, and not only do they understand the language, but they are usually more than happy to talk about it. If you are the non-ill person, it can be a bit of a challenge sometimes feeling like there is always 'someone else in this relationship', a kind of mad Mrs Rochester living in the attic that you can hear padding around once in a while, but is not mentioned. Please consider your relatives; it may feel awkward if you do not create a climate where they can ask or question anything. Try and be as open as possible even if you are naturally one of those types who like to compartmentalize things.

But for new relationships, if you meet someone after diagnosis or treatment, there is one hell of a lot of catch-ups to get through. But it is not all bad: we do not take anything for granted anymore; we have a new perspective which means we often get to the point quicker; we know life does not have to be perfect to be pretty damn good; we have low tolerance for office politics; and we are more honest and less inhibited.

* * *

No doubt, much has been written about the adjustments of returning to work after a long, potentially fatal disease. I will attempt to sum up my experiences in the hope they might make yours seem more normal. I was terrified. I knew I had to walk back into the workplace and face my colleagues and staff who had been reading about my dramas over the last year. Do I brazen it out and walk straight down the centre of the open-plan area and into my little glass office at the end? Or do I attempt to shapeshift, go up the back stairs and magically appear in my office? I went for the shapeshift option and did my best to look like I had been there for ages.

But then what? I needed tea. And things to do. Luckily, I was rescued by my dear PPS Alex, who had laid out a file of things I needed to know, along with a nice cup of tea. The rest of the day I was 'caught' by half the office who wanted to give me a big hug and welcome me back and the other half who avoided any form of contact, eye or otherwise, for fear of catching my embarrassment.

I had outlived my log-ins which all needed resetting. This made me wonder how long I would be able to use the excuse 'I am sorry, I did not receive that email (paper, phone call, and so on)' or claim ignorance for the latest greatest corporate project that was consuming every waking moment of my colleagues' lives.

While I was, of course, grateful to get back to 'normal', I did not feel in the least bit normal and hoped my new perspective on life would last longer than the sell-by date on the canteen's sandwiches.

How do you gradually take management control of a team that has been doing without you for a year? How do you get the right balance of being fit enough to work versus not being quite what you were? As far as priorities were concerned, do you really care about the report deadline or the project milestones? What is the worst thing that can happen?

And how do you take unpopular decisions and give critical feedback when you just want everyone to remember you as lovely in the event of your death?

When I returned to work, I walked slap bang into a restructure request. It was about as far away from my wish list as possible. My creative sixpack was still very firm, and I was looking forward to putting it back to work, coupled with my newfound perspective which I was certain would help me cut through the decision-making process faster than it took me to spell procrastination. Unfortunately, this was not quite the brief awaiting me. No, a year-long absence was 'punished' by requests for a radical restructure. Oh yes, that's head count reduction in case I was not quite clear enough on the objective. There was even talk about another job option for me which was positioned as a little bit less stressful. Not really what I had in mind and so I refused the 'opportunity', but was then left with no other options than to restructure my team. How should I respond when the CEO talks about creating resilience in the team structure? Is it about organizational risk planning?

I spent hours of my precious life worrying about whether they really wanted me back or whether they could not easily kick me out now. I tried to 'act healthy' all the time. I had no colds. No time off. No GP appointments. No protestations of tiredness. No day without makeup. I tried to be even more switched on in case they thought chemo had done in my brain. A casual conversation about the outgoing CEO 'wanting me out' had me very jumpy and bitter for a good week. While I had been fighting for my life, the thought of someone plotting to sideline or remove me filled me with numerous sleepless nights. Until I talked it over with my acupuncturist who said, 'Instead of complaining about the darkness; light a candle', and sent me on my way with renewed vigour.

I was lucky that my company had included a sickness insurance benefit that kicked in after my sick leave, so I was able to cover most of my bills. And they also worked with me to put a reasonably phased 'return to work plan' into action so that I could come back to work with some confidence.

I learnt quite a lot over this period – not only about my rights, but also how to control the flood of information and requests that can follow a return to work after a long absence. At first, it felt like putting my finger in to hold back the Hoover Dam, and it thoroughly tested my new 'zen-ness'.

Your rights at work when you have cancer

1. Cancer is covered by the Disability Discrimination Act (DDA) and Equality Act (EA).

2. That means you are protected and should not be treated any differently just because you have a disability.

3. You can negotiate reasonable changes in your work or workplace. This might be time off work and assurances that your job will still be there when you want to go back. Or it might be more flexible hours if you feel you can still work and want to return to work either during or after treatment.

4. You can negotiate a phased return to work after your treatment and your period of sick leave have finished.

5. Both Acts will give you legal protection if you feel your employer has treated you unfairly.

➡

---

6. Your terms and conditions (and any benefits) you currently get from your employer will remain the same.

7. You do not have to tell your employer you have cancer if you wish, but it will not help you negotiate any changes if that is what you choose.

* * *

I realize now that I have always approached my head like the Victorians did phrenology. There is a space allocated for all the cancer stuff, the work stuff and the family stuff. Which, I assume, means that my cancer, work and family have all remained the same size, and last time I checked everything was in order. The only explanation I could find for this tight squeeze all of a sudden was that work stuff must be growing again in my head.

I had a week when I seriously considered calling in the removal men. I either needed to move to a bigger head, or just be ruthless and learn not to hang on to stuff. Let me tell you that option 2 was by far an easier task.

Going back to work highlighted for me what probably everyone else already knew: I could not chuck out or file stuff. That explained the 11,367 emails in my inbox. The unpacked boxes under my desk from a previous office move three years ago. The two wardrobes at home stuffed full of out-of-season clothes.

I have a bad case of 'just in case' syndrome, and it was starting to eat into my head space. To add to this, I also suffered a little bit from 'man' brain. I go instantly into solving mentality the minute someone hits me with a problem, or challenge, as we are supposed to say these days.

So I trained myself to avoid Twitter, Facebook and text messaging when things got too tight and I felt like running out of space and time. I cut down on phone time and contacting people until I had created more space.

To remind myself how important breathing was – yes, *breathing*, the type you need to be conscious of doing – I set a mobile alarm to go off so that I would not forget to *breathe* every few hours.

* * *

I heard the other day that I now have the same odds of survival as someone throwing himself or herself over the Niagara Falls in a barrel. That's 50 per cent for any of you adrenaline junkies out there!

Is that supposed to reassure me or terrify me? I don't think I feel the same adrenaline rush that someone sitting on top of those waterfalls in a bit of old wood would feel, but there is something of the daredevil in me, and I suppose I do feel some slight rush when my thoughts turn to cheating death.

Everyone reading this who has not had cancer will probably be shaking his or her head now and saying, 'Why is she still going on about death? She has beaten it, hasn't she?'

And that is exactly the thing.

I cannot say that yet. And if a little pre-worrying about it now will help when I need to face it (be it sooner or later, but let's not be coy, one day), then that has got to be a good thing, hasn't it?

So, if I do worry from time to time about the next thing that is going to get me, don't tell me I am being daft or that lightening won't strike twice (tell that to Roy Sullivan, who holds the enviable world record title for being hit by lightening no less than seven times), but just listen for a bit and then ask me if I want a cuppa.

Can I be a contradiction, please? Can I be enthusiastically positive one minute, but think obsessively about the nature of my death the next? Can I laugh and be flippant about the cancer, but be filled with self-righteous indignation when anyone else tells me I have 'beaten it' like crossing a finish line? Can I not want a man, but then go on a date? Can I hate the boredom of cancer and then go back to work and resent not being sat on the sofa?

Cancer makes you contrary. That is a fact.

* * *

Anyone who has stared into the Sly Old Fox's eyes or held his hand and decided 'It's not you, it's me, but I would rather not see you again' feels the born-again fervour. The big question, of course, is how long will it last and will I ever feel I have got over cancer? Will it take another year, five years?

I am not quite ready to call myself a cancer survivor for fear of jinxing it, and yet I do not want to hang on to cancer for a minute longer than necessary. Do I feel the word 'survivor' is accurate or am I pushing my luck too much? Yes, I am in remission. Yes, I am aware of the statistics and possibilities of relapsing. So where does this leave me? Claiming survivorship before the critical five-year mark feels like claiming to be a musician when all you have learnt so far on the piano is chopsticks!

When something changes you as deeply as having cancer does, I am not sure you see things as black or white such as 'life after cancer', but if we need a tag, maybe something like 'life-absorbing cancer' would be closer to the mark –

although I can see that it doesn't roll off the pen or tongue quite as easily.

Someone once told me that you will not forget you had cancer, but there will be a day when the volume dial in your ear is turned down a bit. You will wake up and realize you have not thought about cancer more than a dozen times that day.

Signs that you are getting back to normal

1. Fading memories.
   (You begin to either 'oversell' or 'undersell' your cancer experiences.)

2. Disbelief.
   ('Did we actually go through all that?')

3. Becoming disorganized again (in my case).
   (Time for super organization was over; I did not need to feel the same level of control. I took this as a sign that I was back in the driving seat.)

4. Getting angry at silly things again.

5. Planning a holiday and *not* worrying about the travel insurance.

As Clive James once said, 'Stop worrying ... nobody gets out of this world alive.'

Bits and pieces

My list of lists

My animal metaphors

Sly Old Fox – cancer

The Siamese Cat – Mr H, my bowel surgeon (inscrutable, calm, distant and oriental/mystical)

The Cheshire Cat – Dr W, my oncologist (always smiley)

Felix the Cat – Mr S, my liver surgeon (who has a 'magic bag of tricks')

Banana Giraffe – my cancer persona

Ostrich – me (head in the sand at the beginning)

Rabbit in headlights – me (still)

Hyenas – me and friends laughing in pubs

My A list

Of all the pages I have sweated over in *The C List*, none have reduced me to night-time terrors more than this one for fear of missing someone off this list – or for not doing them justice. You are all very precious to me, and if I have missed anyone, I am deeply sorry. I would say 'Blame the chemo', but that excuse is wearing a little thin now.

Firstly, I would like to dedicate this book to my two utterly brilliant children. Who cared for me, laughed with me and put aside their needs and fears for far too long. Joseph and Lois, you are legends! I am proud beyond belief to be your mum. You are my reason for living, my pride, my joy, my everything.

To Mum and Dad. I have wanted for *nothing*. You have sacrificed so much of your life for me, and I owe you everything. I have never felt anything other than truly spoilt to be your daughter. This book is about hope and positivity and coping with whatever life throws at you, and I can think of no better teachers than my parents who taught me the power of perseverance and love.

To my brother David, my big little brother. I am sorry for being such an attention-seeker. I promise it will stop now! I did not think it was possible, but we have become even closer, and you have taught me so much with your kindness, wicked humour, exceptional generosity and love. I am so proud of being your sis! And to the wonderful Lucie for letting me know how much I was loved and supported.

To my best friend ever and soulmate Jenny Tyler, who kept me sane and my spirits high. And who never missed an opportunity to send me a card or pick-me-up in the post to let me know she was by my side.

To my incredibly close family of cousins, uncles, aunties and then some! Rebecca, you are officially my number one fan on social media and a career in marketing or stand-up comedy beckons! You have made me laugh and cry, and I am incredibly lucky to be your cousin and mate. To Auntie Jane and Uncle Gordon, who have bombarded me with love, funny comments and treats. To my cousins Sharon, Drusilla, Mike and Fenn, Jared, Vicky and Nathan, who have been wonderful and kept me laughing when I was flagging. To Debbie and Andreas, who put on my remission/end of chemo party and refused to take a penny for it. And to Auntie Carol and Uncle Ivor, Rebecca and Hannah, Auntie Di and Uncle Johnny, Uncle Guy and Sandra, even my ex-husband Mike and my treasure of a stepson, Adam.

To Kate Needham for her editorial inspiration when I was flagging, her spirit, love, laughter and especially the red wine out of taps at Table 8 during chemo. I owe you so much more than you in your humble way ever accepted.

To Andy Blackford for pushing me into writing this in the first place and supplying the title, the regular lunches, advice on meditation and hours of belly laughs.

To Alison Bateman, who laid down the original challenge and motivated me weekly.

To my dearest friends Jo and Kim P, who did a million acts of kindness and still thought they were doing nothing (Jo, I am looking at you!). To Di and Stu, who showered me with love, gave me more food than I could eat and took me into their home when I might have felt isolated or blue. To Julie and Richard for not only giving me the party of a lifetime, but also for being my (and especially Lois's) second family. To my old mate Tina for reminding me that I am still normal, and to Alex for keeping all the stress she could off me and being my one and only PPS!

To my children's best friends: Livvy, who I would adopt in a heartbeat – I cannot thank you enough for being there for Lois; Matthew for being there for Joseph when he was alone and needed a mate; Carys, Rosie and Oli for making Lois laugh and her mum Romi for being calm and intuitive.

And most of all to Lauren Pettitt, who has shown love and maturity beyond her years and supported Joseph, Lois *and* me throughout all this. I owe her eternal love and thanks. She has been, and continues to be, a massive help to us all.

To Mum and Dad's big supporter, Andrew, who phoned daily with love and encouragement.

To Mary Y and Kathy H, who set me straight from the beginning and let me know there was hope. And phoned me regularly just when I needed a pep talk.

To Liz for making me laugh out loud at cancer and helping me see our surgeon Mr H in a different light.

To Mindy for showing me courage and spirit.

And to all my friends and colleagues and those who have kindly supported me on with phone calls, blogs and online: Tracy T, Claire S, Liz W, Bex, Elice, Bruce, Wendy, Mark S, Nick M, Simon C, Ronnie and Kathy, Caroline, Nicole and Glen, Sona, Anna, Liz, Greg, Shelley, Leah, Sally, John P, Rachel and Simon, Dave C, Grant, Tina S, Chris S, Siobhan, Pamela, Sandra B, Joe and Aileen, Sally and Wayne, Leanda and Matt, Jane W, Colin and Rachel, David W and Sue H.

To my fellow online friends and fighters who inspire me, some still battling, some sadly not: Ruthie Dunn, Hayley, Rachel (Rach) and Rachael, Hannah (SMG), Joanne (Boho), Paul (Coxio), Jill (Faraway), Tony L, Adrian (smile a mile), Alison S, Hazel, Lorna, Lisa Lynch, John A, Charley, Mark Mcstillhere, Eddie S, Gina P and Gina and Steve, Mark Flannagan, Peter and Sheila, Clint, Sian B, Nellyjuke, Chris (subtitles), Laura (paperdollybird) and her amazing mum Lesley, Ann C, Helen C, Katie and Stuart, Gail A, Julie S, Daf J, Jane B, Rita D, Rebekah HB and Rebecca Joyce, Anne C (sisteranne), Lindsay and Neil.

To Bowel Cancer UK and Beating Bowel Cancer for all your support, knowledge and friendship. Especially Deborah Alsina, who is a legend.

To my nutritionist Juliet Haywood and my acupuncturist David Wilson for making me look and feel so well.

To my agent, Clare Hulton, for believing in me.

To Mr H, my bowel surgeon, Mr S, my liver surgeon 1, Mr S, my liver surgeon 2, and Dr W, my oncologist (please forgive me for the animal metaphors), for none other than saving my life, and Lesley for being so compassionate.

To all my new friends at the church, too numerous to mention.

And, finally, I am thrilled to say, to John Haynes, who I met after this book was finished when I was in remission. John has captured my heart and stayed through everything that has been thrown at me since, showing gentleness, compassion and extreme love. He is very precious and we are getting married. You can all breathe a sigh of relief now!

Postscript

The PS bit

I have been obsessing about whether to add this postscript. Despite not being a 'neat freak', I did hope this book would end with remission and normality. But … in the space in between sending the script to my publisher and them getting round to printing it, there was a bit of a setback.

I feel like apologizing for tucking this in unannounced just when you were no doubt expecting the happy and tidy ending. But I would feel like I was holding out on you by *not* squeezing in this update. And anyway, it all ends well, so I feel I should be up front.

So having gone round the houses enough now to make even Kirsty Allsop dizzy, here it is …

The cancer came back. The pain in my bum that I was most worried about the last few months did not turn out to be cancer. But the dull ache in my right-hand side and my shoulders did. No, the Sly Old Fox did not naff off as it had promised. It hid and waited until my life was getting pretty near perfect again and then decided to come back. This time, again in my liver.

I had rehearsed this day enough times to reduce the shock impact, but I must admit that I was not ready for the huge sense of disappointment of having done everything I could do (with my dad's constant supplies of pills, wheatgrass juice, vitamin D, acupuncture and exercise) to stop this. Yet, here we were again, facing more treatment and having conversations with men who spend their daylight hours cutting bits out of your body (I shudder to think what they get up to during the night).

But in among the lows, I have had, and will continue to have, the most incredible highs. I have a new man, John. He turned up totally unexpected a short while ago and is the kindest, strongest and most loving man I have ever had the pleasure of going out with. Somehow he has taken each and every knock I have thrown his way these past couple of months, culminating with this humdinger, with the best grace, humour, fortitude and, most importantly, love.

Once Mr H, the Siamese Cat, phoned me to tell me on the same day of my CT scan (never a good sign!) that there were a couple of spots on my liver which needed investigating, I was thrown back into cancer speak. We had another MRI scan to check it was cancer (it was), but the scariest appointment was having another PET CT scan to see if there were any other cancerous 'hot spots' lurking around. My doctor, the 'normal' one who still gives me treats like prescriptions and cervical smear tests (not the one that nukes me or the one that cuts bits of me out), well, she explained that the PET CT scan would check to see how the cancerous cells are behaving and how fast they are turning over. It would also check for any other sites of cancer gobbling glucose behaving badly that might scupper any plans for surgery. I would be injected with heavy metals, made to wee in a special loo and be restricted from kissing babies or pregnant women. And then after 90 minutes when they hoped I would sit still and wait for the radiation to circulate throughout my body, I was to lie down in the PET scanner with my hands above my head in the diving position and not move a muscle for 45 minutes. Sounds good to you? Yes, to me, too …

After a terrifying wait I was treated to the news that my cancer, on its return visit, was definitely confined to my liver. And as far as my oncologist would commit himself, just in the left lobe, segments two and three. Okay, he would not say, 'For sure, it's definitely *not* in the right lobe.' But no one can see anything yet. Apparently, once you have had secondary cancer, you do not hear phrases like 'It's not there' or 'It's all gone', only 'We can't see anything' or 'There is no evidence' … Still, it was the best sentence I had heard since the cancer returned.

Things then moved quite quickly, and within a few weeks I had another J0310. For those of you about to complain 'They don't sell that in my local', it is actually medical code for a liver tumour removal together with a chunk of liver on the side. It finally went ahead on July 22 at the Churchill Hospital, where I had to do a quick mental adjustment, remove it from my 'been there, done that' filing space in my brain and re-file it into my 'here we go again' box.

To mix it up a bit this time, it was the other lobe (left one) that was being hacked off, also known as the pointy end of the iron/liver. I was checked into a slightly different room two doors down from my last liver resection and also changed surgeons mid consultation! My 'old' one, Felix the Cat, was on call that day, but said he would try to pop in for a look. The way I used to pop in as an optional attendee in random meetings, where I could sit quite comfortably in the knowledge that I would have no actions and be happily unaccountable.

I realize that having liver surgery twice may not sound like a treat to those of you reading without squatters in your liver, but for those of us with, it is, indeed. My oncologist said we would not be sitting here contemplating another surgery as recently as four years previously. If that is not enough to freeze-dry your bones, only about 20 per cent of all liver tumours are considered removable by surgery. So to fall into this camp twice is considered a great blessing. Although newer treatments such as RFA, SIRT and cyber knife are also proving to be really successful, it is nice to know there is still something up my surgeon's sleeve should it come back again.

I guess if there is any point at all of this update, it is to say that treatment options and longer-term survivability are in a much better place now than ever before, but you need to know your options, push for answers and do not take a 'no', ever. Look at me: I am, with the grace of God, living proof.

After a shaky start where our respective sense of humours looked on with mutual horror – his dry as a bone and mine a nervous stream of nonsense – my new surgeon, another Mr S (I have not quite decided on his nickname), was outrageously awesome and totally charmed me into submission. I did not even protest when, the morning after the operation, he said, 'What are you still doing lazing about in bed? Stop treating this place like your hotel!' I even smiled with him when he laughed out loud after lifting my gown to reveal the purple patchwork quilt that used to be called my stomach. And when he denied 'touching my bowels' and rendering them catatonic, I found his offer of 'putting some dynamite up me' strangely charming.

I will gloss over the operation and subsequent stay in hospital and will only say that it was bad enough to cash in my holiday voucher and leave for saner places before the expiry date. But you will be delighted to know that my new surgeon has offered me my operation on film, saying, 'I wouldn't watch it with your hand in the popcorn bucket if I were you, but I figured, as you never stop asking me questions and telling me how to do my job, you might be interested in seeing your textbook operation!'

It is difficult to know what to say that has not been said before. It is certainly more boring the second time around when you completely lose any morbid fascination you may previously have had. But I do have a few titbits for you!

1. A liver drain is called a Robinson drain, or a Mrs Robinson drain if, like me, you are now older than your surgeon.

2. Phlebotomists (vampires) now have to drag around a WOW or a COW. It stands for 'working on wheels' or 'computer on wheels' and holds your EPR or electronic patient record, but is very cumbersome. So much so that they arrived on day 1 and I never saw them again.

3. The room where they put you to sleep has a tray full of 'bear huggers'. Isn't that nice?

4. The only bit of the operation that is pleasant is the GA bit, so make sure you ask to be counted down from ten so that you can jolly well enjoy it. Mine took me on a very long, slow trip and it was delicious.

5. Surgeons wind you up on day 2. I think it is part of the recovery programme.

6. If, like me, your veins are shut for business, a nice anaesthetist can put in a central line into your neck, a bit like a temporary PICC line that makes countless injections and drips painless.

7. IV paracetamol is much more effective (don't ask me why) than tablets, but costs more, so you have to stare down the nurse and growl a bit.

8. The anti-sickness drug Cyclizine, applied as an IV when under the influence of morphine, will blow your head clean

off for two hours. Well, it did mine and was, again, jolly nice. But once I mentioned this to the nursing staff, I was banned from any more ...

There is time for just one final update! Great news is I had clear margins again from the liver operation. So the surgery was a success. But ...

I was getting increasingly nervous of going within sniffing distance of a hospital. Every time I as much sneezed near one, I seemed to get more holes in my body. Or as John said to me after all this kicked off again, 'They might as well put a zip in it.'

My recovery from my second liver op was slightly more complicated than before: I suffered an infection in my main exit wound (a seroma, apparently, a pocket of clear serous fluid) and a lump appeared where my liver drain was. While we were still working out if it was a haematoma (a delicious collection of blood) or a hernia, the infection instead of dying down revved up and demanded more attention than I was giving it.

So just for a change, I was readmitted to hospital and subjected to repeated tests (some we will never understand were quite necessary, thank you very much indeed!) and others which seemed a little over the top, X-rays at 2.30am and CT scans. Happily, this resulted in my being plugged into the hardcore antibiotics that I needed to sort out the infection – and a promise to finally get this infection under control.

After many hours on a trolley in the surgical assessment ward (also known as the ward where s/he who cries loudest gets the first bed), I was transferred to a nice quiet room as payment for my patience and met David Bailey. Well, I met one of the David Baileys. My male tattooed nurse tried to get into *The Guinness Book of Records* by taking part in a stunt to get over 126 David Baileys together in one place. I think he was about three David's short, so didn't make it.

Then followed a procession of doctors who wanted to have a gander at my scars and lumps and bumps and, noticing the haematoma/hernia, poked it very hard until it popped. I suppose it was lucky (although it did not appear so at the time) that this set off one of my extremely painful bowel spasms that I have been having since the liver surgery (it is put down to scar tissue). This time, David Bailey was on hand to witness and he did not like it one bit. He pumped me full of Tramadol and, when this did not touch the sides, squirted morphine into my mouth before I could tell him he would regret it later when he came to clear up the bathroom or 'barf room' as it became known.

My surgeon who got wind of this came to see me and told me in a stern voice that I was going to have an operation to fix the small bowel hernia and stop the kink in my bowel and that it was going to be that same evening. No, thank you, he really was not interested to hear that I was going to Cornwall on Thursday for a week's holiday …

So yes, another op and yet more holes in an already holey tummy, but I am feeling great and relieved it is all over, finally. Please!

'Didn't dating used to be a lot easier than this?' said John wistfully as he wheeled me out of the John Radcliffe into his car as we made our escape.

Therefore do not worry about tomorrow, for tomorrow will worry about itself. Each day has enough trouble of its own.

Matthew 6:34